THE OCINATOR

# RESTAURANT DIET:

# 1,000+

# HEALTHY MENU ITEMS

NICO CHAVANDO

Restaurants reserve the right to change their menus at any time.

Please note that *The Ocinator Restaurant Diet* does not constitute medical advice, and you should consult with your healthcare professional before making any changes to your diet.

ISBN-13: 978-1-7329251-0-6

Available in E-Book.

# Restaurants by Cuisine

**Asian**
Benihana
Panda Express
Pei Wei Asian Diner
P.F. Chang's
Poke (General)

**Mexican**
Chili's Grill & Bar
Chipotle
Chuy's
El Pollo Loco
On The Border
Pollo Tropical
Taco Bell
Taco Cabana
Taco John's

**Italian**
California Pizza Kitchen
Carraba's Italian Grill
Cicis Pizza
Domino's
Jet's Pizza
Maggiano's Little Italy
Olive Garden
Papa John's

# Restaurants by Menu Item

**Bowls**
BJ's Restaurant & Brewhouse
Bob Evans (fish)
California Pizza Kitchen
Chipotle
El Pollo Loco
First Watch
Jamba Juice
Moe's Southwest Grill
Olive Garden
On the Border Mexican Grill & Cantina
P.F. Chang's
Pollo Tropical
Qdoba
Taco Bell
Taco Cabana
Tropical Smoothie Café
Yard House
Zoës

**Eggs**
Bob Evans
Chick-fil-A
Corner Bakery Cafe
Cracker Barrel Old Country Store
Denny's
First Watch
IHOP
O'Charley's
Panera Bread

**Eggs (cont.)**
Perkins Restaurant & Bakery
Taco Cabana
Taco John's
The Cheesecake Factory
Village Inn
Waffle House

**Grilled Chicken Sandwiches**
Bar Louie
Burger King
Carl's Jr.
Carraba's Italian Grill
Cheddar's Scratch Kitchen
Corner Bakery Cafe
Cracker Barrel Old Country Store
Culver's
Dairy Queen
Dave and Buster's
Denny's
Firehouse Subs
Freddy's Frozen Custard and Steakburgers
Hardee's
Hungry Howie's
Longhorn Steakhouse
McDonald's
Ruby Tuesday
Steak 'n Shake

**Pasta**
Maggiano's
Olive Garden

**Pizza**
Bertucci's

**Poke**
P.F. Chang's
Poke (General)
Yard House

**Smoothies**
Jamba Juice
Tropical Smoothie Café

**Tacos**
Chuy's
El Pollo Loco
Moe's Southwest Grill
On The Border Mexican Grill & Cantina
Qdoba
Red Lobster (fish & chicken)
Taco Cabana
Taco John's
The Cheesecake Factory

# Table of Contents

# About the Author

Nico Chavando is the founder of Ocinator.com and the Ocinator Fitness Program. He obtained his Product Design Degree from Stanford University. There, he experimented with different approaches to being fit and healthy long-term.

Nico used his background in Design Thinking to identify a problem affecting 40% of the population, obesity and obesity-related diseases, and to offer an attainable, easy solution. While trendy diets and workout programs grow in popularity, the obesity rate is not decreasing. In fact, obesity-related conditions like heart disease, stroke, type 2 diabetes, and certain types of cancer continue to be some of the leading causes of preventable premature death.

Nico found that many current diets make people think that eating healthily involves counting calories, limiting food consumption, complicated meal preparation, avoiding good protein sources, and/or eliminating carbs. Unfortunately, these common misconceptions about healthy eating lead some to adopt unrealistic and possibly harmful diets. These painful diets rely on dramatic changes of habits and often cause constant feelings of hunger, decreased mental sharpness, and negative changes in mood including crankiness, hostility, and depression.

1 in 3 Americans eats out on any given day, either for work or social reasons, because we are busy, do not like to cook, or just because we prefer eating out! Many of us are concerned with our weight and overall health and would like to eat healthy foods at restaurants, but end up ordering unhealthy menu items. This is because we either do not know how to modify restaurant orders to make them

healthy, or because tweaking orders is a hassle to think about when we are in a rush.

Helping restaurant-goers eat a sound meal is a need that was largely unmet by diet books… until now.

We need a quick and easy guide to help us eat in a healthy way and feel good without becoming chefs. So, Nico created *The Ocinator Restaurant Diet*. With over 1,000 healthy menu options, this book helps busy folks like you to eat on the go, healthily, and without the pain that many other diets produce. It is an ongoing solution to promote long-term health.

*The Ocinator Restaurant Diet* has helped many people of all ages eat healthily every day and be amazed at the results. You can have the strength, energy, and positivity provided by delicious, healthy food and be fit! Nico hopes this guide will help you and many more feel great long-term too.

# Introduction

Busy and want something quick to eat? Don't like to cook? Traveling? Or just love eating out? *The Ocinator Restaurant Diet* was designed to show you exactly how to choose healthy menu options at the most popular chain restaurants in the U.S.

Learn how to eat healthily without starving yourself or counting calories!

The latest medical research shows that "a calorie is not a calorie," meaning that in a healthy lifestyle the quality of the food eaten matters more than the quantity of food eaten. Common sense tells us that it is healthier to eat 100 calories of vegetables than 100 calories of chocolate cake.

*The Ocinator Restaurant Diet* lists healthy food you can eat at restaurants to help you lose weight the simple way, without the pain of starvation of no-carb diets.

The following pages help explain how *The Ocinator Restaurant Diet* is effective and why you will benefit from the following suggestions.

<u>Keys to Remember</u>

1. Small changes make a huge difference.
2. Be brave.
3. Be consistent.
4. Think results and after-effects… to say no to junk food now.

**1. Small changes make a huge difference.**

It might seem like the difference between white bread and whole grain bread, water and lemonade, dressing and no dressing, are of little significance. False. These small changes are what allow you to lose fat without spending all day doing cardio.

Know that the small changes you make add up and help sculpt an amazing body through a realistic and physically painless process. Our good small choices add up for the better!

**2. Be brave.**

Do not be afraid to ask servers to modify menu options! You are paying for the food which directly affects how healthy you look and feel. Be brave and ask for the food you need to succeed.

**3. Be consistent.**

Do not take days off. Of course, at first it may be difficult to give up certain things like white bread, dressing, cheese, sugary foods, and butter. Ease off these foods, and notice how your taste buds improve and how great you look and feel.

**4. Think results and after-effects... to say no to junk food now.**

When resisting the temptation to eat unhealthy food, think about how unhealthy junk food makes you feel after you eat it. The healthier you eat, the more you will be able to notice how badly junk food makes the body feel. Thinking about how badly junk food makes your body feel can help stop you from eating junk food in the first place.

## General Healthy Food Guidelines

**Stay away from refined grains.**

The prominent advice in medicine today indicates how to

lose weight in a healthy way: stay away from products with *refined grain* and products with added sugar. Also, eat lots of vegetables. The key: *refined grain* carbs are bad. On the other hand, *whole grain* carbs are good.

*Refined grain* carbs are unhealthy because they have been stripped of the nutrients that whole grains have. But because *whole grain* carbs have those nutrients, they are good for you.

Studies have shown that not eating whole grain carbs could lead to: poorer memory-based task performance, bad breath, and increased anger, depression, anxiety, irritability, and hostility.

On the other hand, eating whole grain carbs could lead to positive effects by allowing the soluble fiber, found in whole grain carbs, to:

- Decrease LDL (bad) cholesterol
- Increase good HDL cholesterol
- Increase dietary fiber
- Help promote fat loss
- Prevent fat gain
- Lower the risk of diabetes

*Refined grains* do not provide these potential benefits.

**Stay away from products with added sugar and artificial sweeteners.**

The more you stay away from products with added sugar, the sweeter naturally sweet food, like fruit, will taste!

Stay away from: soda, most desserts, dressings, syrups, jams, jellies, etc. Instead, try eating naturally sweet food like fruit.

Look out for hidden sugars and additives. For example, dressing contains too much added sugar as well as saturated fat and sodium that can lead to increased body fat and feelings of hunger.

Research changes regarding the side effects of artificial sweeteners, so it is best to avoid them.

Again, small changes like eating fruit and getting rid of salad dressing add up and make a huge difference!

**Balance your meats.**

Though this book lists beef menu options, it is not a free pass to eat beef during every meal. Try eating mostly chicken and fish. Consuming too much red meat can be unhealthy.

**Eat lots of vegetables.**

We all know the many benefits of eating most vegetables! Let's have more fiber and freshness.

Overall Fitness

*The Ocinator Restaurant Diet* is intended to help users lose body fat. To help you sculpt abs and other muscles, we recommend the Ocinator Fitness Program as the ideal companion to this book. Ocinator workouts are simple and do not aim for sweat and exhaustion.

On the contrary, Ocinator workouts were designed to minimize workout time (20 minutes/day) and pain so that users can realistically maintain results and a positive long-term change in fitness lifestyle. See Ocinator.com for more details.

Both *The Ocinator Restaurant Diet* and Ocinator Fitness aim to make obtaining and maintaining long-term fitness results simple and realistic.

Now… it's time to enjoy all your new restaurant menu options and feel great!

## General Ordering Guidelines

Be comfortable asking for:

- Whole grains, brown rice - instead of white/refined carbs*
- Food that is steamed, baked/grilled with no/minimal oil
- Lemon slices, vinegar, mustard, guacamole/avocados, or fresh salsa, pepper and other herbs - instead of dressings, condiments and sauces that contain extra oils/fats

*Including free appetizers

## General Cuisine Guidelines

### Mexican

Stay away from: chips, cheese, Mexican rice, white flour tortillas, and hard-shell (fried) tortillas.
Choose soft corn tortillas or brown rice instead.

### Italian

Stay away from: white flour (bread, pizza dough, pasta dough) and cheese.
Choose whole wheat options.

### Asian

Stay away from: stir fry (ask for food to be cooked with little to no oil), refined grain (white rice and noodles), butter (on meat, especially), and sauce.
Choose steamed foods, brown rice, and ginger and pepper.

### American

Stay away from: fried food, cheese, sauce, dressing/vinaigrette, and white bread/buns (including free appetizers).

Choose grilled and whole wheat options.

*Stick to water or low-fat milk, unless we list drink items like healthy smoothies. (No soda, juice, or alcohol.)

# Restaurant Menu Items With Healthy Tweaks

# Applebee's

Drink: Water

## Appetizers

- House Salad

  *without: cheese, croutons, and dressing*
- Chicken Tortilla Soup

  *without: tortilla strips and cheese*
- Tomato Basil

  *without: croutons and cheese*

## Sides/Extras

- Baked Potato

  *without: butter, sour cream, cheese, bacon, etc.*
- Steamed Broccoli

## Steaks & Ribs

- 6 oz. or 8 oz. Top Sirloin

  *without: butter. see above for sides/extras*

## Chicken

- Cedar Grilled Lemon Chicken

  *without: cranberry-pecan rice (quinoa instead) and vinaigrette/dressing (ask for lemon slices instead)*

## Salads

*instead of dressing, ask for: lemon, pepper, vinegar, guacamole/avocados, or fresh salsa*

- Southwest Steak Salad

  *without: chimichurri, cheese, tortilla strips, and ranch*
- Grilled Chicken Salad

  *without: cheese and dressing*

## Seafood

- Cedar Salmon

  *without: maple mustard glaze. see above for sides/extras*

# Applebee's (2)

Drink: Water

## Sandwiches

- Clubhouse Grille
  *without: potato bread (instead, whole wheat/grain bread or lettuce bun)*
  *without: bacon, cheese, honey bbq, mayo, and fries*

## Burgers

Classic Burger
*without: white bread bun (instead, whole wheat/grain bread or lettuce bun), cheese, sauce, pickles, and fries*

# Arby's

Drink: Water

## Entrée

- Turkey Avocado Club
  *without: honey wheat bread (lettuce bun instead), bacon, and mayo*
- Roast Turkey Farmhouse Salad
  *without: honey wheat bread, bacon, and cheese*
- Roast Turkey Wrap
  *without: white flour wrap (wheat grain wrap instead), bacon, cheese, mayonnaise, and ranch*

## Sides

- Chopped Side Salad
  *without: cheese, croutons, and dressing*

# Au Bon Pain

Drink: Water

## Soups

- 12 Veggie
- Vegetable Beef & Barley

## Sandwiches

- Turkey Sandwich
  *without: Swiss cheese and honey pecan spread*
- Black Angus Roast Beef Sandwich
  *without: cheddar and dijonnaise*

## Wraps

- Napa Chicken With Avocado
  *without: white flour wrap (whole wheat wrap instead), aïoli, and lemon shallot vinaigrette*
- Harvest Turkey
  *without: mayo and cheddar*

## Salads

*instead of dressing, ask for: lemon, pepper, vinegar, guacamole/avocados, or fresh salsa*

- Chicken Cobb with Avocado
  *without: bacon*
- Vegetarian Deluxe
- Harvest Turkey
  *without: goat cheese*

# Bar Louie

Drink: Water

Sandwiches

- California Chicken Club
  *without: bacon, pepper jack, and ranch. with side of fruit or salad without dressing, cheese, and croutons*

Burgers

- Ask for a burger on whole grain bread with just the beef patty, tomato, and lettuce (without cheese, sauce, etc.)

# Benihana

Drink: Water

<u>Entrées</u>

- Hibachi Chicken
  *without: butter on chicken and vegetables*
- Hibachi Shrimp
  *without: butter on shrimp and vegetables*
- Filet Mignon
  *without: butter on filet mignon and vegetables*
- Hibachi Steak
  *without: butter on steak and vegetables*
- Beef Julienne
  *without: butter on beef and vegetables*

<u>Sides</u>

- Benihana Salad
  *without: dressing. with vinegar instead*
- Brown Rice
- Miso Soup

# Bertucci's

Drink: Water

## Brick Oven Pizzas

Multigrain Dough

+ *sliced cherry peppers, broccoli, mushrooms, bell peppers, onions, diced plum tomatoes, sliced tomatoes, spinach, and/or arugula*

+ (optional) *roasted garlic, roasted black olives, roasted zucchini, roasted peppers, roasted artichokes, roasted eggplant, and/or roasted button mushrooms*

+ (optional) *red wine vinegar*

+ (optional) *chicken, meatballs, and/or rosemary ham*

*without: cheese, bacon, pepperoni, sauce, and dressing*

## Pasta Classics

- Spaghetti & Polpette (Meatballs)
  *without: white flour pasta (whole wheat linguine instead) and cheese*
- Chicken Domani (with Grilled Chicken substitute)
  *without: white flour pasta (whole wheat linguine instead), cheese, and white wine sauce (pomodoro instead)*
- Rigatoni, Broccoli, and Chicken (with Grilled Chicken substitute)
  *without: white flour pasta (whole wheat linguine instead), cheese, sautéed breaded chicken (grilled chicken instead), white wine sauce (pomodoro instead)*
- Rigatoni, Broccoli, and Shrimp (with Grilled Shrimp)
  *without: white flour pasta (whole wheat linguine instead), cheese, and white wine or lemon-garlic cream sauce (pomodoro instead)*

## Soups

- Minestrone
  *without: cheese*
- Lentil Soup
  *without: caramelized onions, sautéed garlic, evoo, balsamic vinegar, and hand-chopped parsley*

# Bertucci's (2)

Drink: Water

## Starters

- Polpette (Meatballs)
  *without: cheese*
- Antipasto
  *without: mozzarella, balsamic fig drizzle, pecorino romano, salami, stuffed green olives with grilled prosciutto rolled around fresh mozzarella, and grilled rosemary focaccia*

## Salads

*instead of dressing, ask for: lemon, pepper, vinegar, guacamole/avocados, or fresh salsa*

- Farmhouse Salad (with Grilled Shrimp, Grilled Chicken, or Grilled Salmon)
  *without: cheese, pepperoni, balsamic fig glaze, and vinaigrette/dressing*
- Shrimp & Spinach Gorgonzola Salad (with Grilled Shrimp, Grilled Chicken, or Grilled Salmon)
  *without: cheese and vinaigrette/dressing*
- Insalata
  *without: cheese and vinaigrette/dressing*
- Shrimp Mediterraneo Salad (with Grilled Shrimp, Grilled Chicken, or Grilled Salmon)
  *without: cheese and vinaigrette/dressing*
- Grilled Chicken Caesar Salad
  *without: cheese, croutons, and vinaigrette/dressing*
- Baby Arugula & Grilled Chicken
  *without: vinaigrette/dressing*

## Specialty Entrées

- Bistecca
  *without: sautéed spinach (grilled instead) and Marsala sauce (pomodoro instead)*
- Roasted Eggplant Pomodoro
  *without: spaghetti (whole grain linguine instead) and mozzarella*

# Bertucci's (3)

Drink: Water

<u>Seafood Entrées</u>

- Salmon
  *without: sautéed spinach (grilled or cooked with little to no oil instead). ask for potatoes to be grilled or cooked without oil*
- Cod Limone
  *without: cheese and angel hair pasta (whole wheat linguine instead)*

<u>Chicken Entrées</u>

- Chicken Piccata
  *without: sautéed breaded chicken (grilled chicken instead), egg fettuccine (whole wheat linguine instead), white wine sauce (pomodoro instead), and cheese*
- Chicken Anna Maria
  *without: sautéed breaded chicken (grilled chicken instead), egg fettuccine (whole wheat linguine instead), and cream sauce (pomodoro instead)*
- Chicken Marsala
  *without: Marsala wine sauce (pomodoro instead), spaghetti (whole wheat linguine instead), and cheese. ask for potatoes to be cooked with little to no oil*

Remember:
**Small changes make a huge difference.**
Know that the small changes you make add up and help sculpt an amazing body through a realistic and physically painless process. Our small choices add up for the better!

# BJ's Restaurant & Brewhouse

Drink: Water

## Entrées

- Enlightened Chicken Quinoa Bowl
  *ask for steamed, not sautéed, vegetables and very little olive oil*
- Enlightened Lemon Thyme Chicken
  *ask for steamed, not sautéed, vegetables*
  *without lemon thyme sauce*
- Enlightened Fire-Roasted Barbacoa Chicken
  *without: feta cheese and crema*
- House Top Sirloin
  *with two of the following sides: asparagus (steamed), black beans, bowl of soup, salad (no cheese and dressing), broccoli (steamed), quinoa*
- BJ's Classic Rib-Eye
  *with two of the following sides: asparagus (steamed), black beans, bowl of soup, salad (no cheese and dressing), broccoli (steamed), quinoa*

## Soups

- Chicken Tortilla Soup
  *without: tortilla strips (usually fried). ask for soft corn tortillas instead, if available*
- Tomato Bisque
  *without croutons*

## Salads

*instead of dressing, ask for: lemon, pepper, vinegar, guacamole/avocados, or fresh salsa*

- House Salad
  *without: Parmesan cheese and croutons*

# Bob Evans

Drink: Water

## Entrées

- Grilled Chicken Breast
  *without white bread. see below for sides*
- Grilled Salmon
  *without white bread. see below for sides*
- USDA Choice Sirloin
  *without white bread. see below for sides*
- Handcrafted Deli Turkey Sandwich
  *without: marble wheat bread (whole wheat/grain bread or lettuce bun instead), Swiss cheese, and mayo. instead of fries, see below for healthy sides*

## Family Meals

- Grilled Chicken Breasts
  *with two of the following sides: asparagus (steamed), black beans, bowl of soup, salad (no cheese and dressing), broccoli (steamed), quinoa*

## Soups

- Chicken & Noodles
  *without: noodles*
- Hearty Beef Vegetable Soup

## Sides

- Seasonal Fresh Fruit
- Farmhouse Garden Salad
  *without: tortilla strips, cheddar cheese, and dressing*

# Bob Evans (2)

Drink: Water

<u>Breakfast</u>

*ask for food to be cooked without butter and with little to no oil*

- Rise & Shine
  *with ham and fruit (as a side) and more fruit instead of white bread (get whole wheat/grain bread if available) or potatoes cooked with little to no oil*
  *without: white bread, biscuits, hash browns, fries, and grits*
- Sirloin Steak & Farm Fresh Eggs
  *with ham and fruit (as a side) and more fruit instead of white bread (get whole wheat/grain bread if available) or potatoes cooked with little to no oil*
  *without: white bread, biscuits, hash browns, fries, and grits*

<u>Salads</u>

*instead of dressing, ask for: lemon, pepper, vinegar, guacamole/avocados, or fresh salsa*

- Wildfire Chicken Salad
  *without: tortilla strips, cheddar cheese, and dressing*
- Cranberry Pecan Chicken Salad
  *without: bacon, bleu cheese, and dressing*
- Cobb Salad
  *without: bacon, bleu cheese, and dressing*

Remember:
The latest medical research shows that "a calorie is not a calorie," meaning that in a healthy lifestyle the quality of the food eaten matters more than the quantity of food eaten. Common sense tells us that it is healthier to eat 100 calories of vegetables than 100 calories of chocolate cake.

# Bonefish Grill

Drink: Water

Dinner

- Chilean Sea Bass
  *without: butter or sauce*
- Atlantic Salmon
  *without: butter or sauce*
- Ahi Tuna Steak
  *without: butter or sauce*
- Rainbow Tuna
  *without: butter or sauce*
- Filet Mignon
  *without: butter*
- Bone-In Ribeye Steak
  *without: butter*
- Sirloin Steak
  *without: butter*
- Lily's Chicken
  *without: goat cheese and lemon basil sauce*
- Dynamite-Style Shrimp
  *without: aïoli and feta cheese*
- Cold Water Lobster Tails
  *without: butter*

Salads

*instead of dressing, ask for: lemon, pepper, vinegar, guacamole/avocados, or fresh salsa*

- Bonefish Cobb Salad
  *without: blue cheese, bacon, and ranch*
- Bonefish House Salad
  *without: citrus herb vinaigrette*
- Grilled Salmon Superfood Salad
  *without: feta, vinaigrette, and citrus aïoli*

# Boston Market

Drink: Water

Entrées

- Rotisserie Chicken (Half Chicken, Quarter White, or Three-Piece Dark)
  *see below for sides*
- Rotisserie Turkey Breast
  *see below for sides*

Soups

- Rotisserie Chicken Soups
  *without noodles*

Salads

*instead of dressing, ask for: lemon, pepper, vinegar, guacamole/avocados, or fresh salsa*

- House Salad
  *without: Parmesan cheese and croutons*

Sides

- Fresh Steamed Vegetables
- Salad
  *without: dressing and cheese*

# Buffalo Wild Wings

Drink: Water

<u>Salads</u>

*instead of dressing, ask for: lemon, pepper, vinegar, guacamole/avocados, or fresh salsa*

- Santa Fe Salad (Grilled Chicken)
  *without: cheese, tortilla strips, ranch, and flour tortillas (instead, get soft corn tortillas if available)*
- Garden Chicken Salad (Grilled Chicken)
  *without: Parmesan, croutons, vinaigrette, and toast*
- Side Salad
  *without: Parmesan, croutons, vinaigrette, and toast*

<u>Tenders</u>

- Naked Tenders
  *without: sauce and fries (ask for a salad without dressing as a substitute for fries)*

# Burger King

Drink: Water

<u>Sandwiches</u>

- Grilled Chicken Sandwich
  *without: white bread bun (instead, lettuce bun or whole wheat bun if available) and mayo*
  Why not the potato bun? It contains refined flour, which contributes to weight gain.

<u>Salads</u>

*instead of dressing, ask for: lemon, pepper, vinegar, guacamole/avocados, or fresh salsa*

- Chicken Garden Salad
  *without: croutons, cheese, and dressing/vinaigrette*
- Garden Side Salad
  *without: croutons, cheese, and dressing/vinaigrette*

# California Pizza Kitchen

Drink: Water

## Soups

- Sedona Tortilla
  *without: tortilla strips (unless they are baked, not fried). instead, get soft corn tortillas if available*

## Power Bowls

- Banh Mi Bowl
  *without vinaigrette*
- Santa Fe Bowl
  *without ranch*

## Salads

*instead of dressing, ask for: lemon, pepper, vinegar, guacamole/avocados, or fresh salsa*

- Roasted Veggie (Grilled Chicken or Shrimp)
  *without vinaigrette*
- Waldorf Chicken
  *without: vinaigrette and candied walnuts*
- California Cobb
  *without: bacon and dressing*
- Quinoa + Arugula
  *without: feta and vinaigrette*

## Main Plates

- Hearth-Roasted Halibut
  *without creamy farro*
- Cedar Plank Salmon
  *without feta*

*Note: Cauliflower pizza dough is unhealthy, as it contains mozzarella cheese*

# Captain D's Seafood Kitchen

Drink: Water

<u>Salads</u>

*instead of dressing, ask for: lemon, pepper, vinegar, guacamole/avocados, or fresh salsa*

- Wild Alaskan Salmon Salad
  *without: dressing and breadstick*

<u>Sides</u>

- Side Salad
  *without dressing*
- Broccoli
  *without feta*
- Baked Potato
  *without: butter and sour cream*
- Corn
  *without butter*

<u>Grilled Meals</u>

*for each of the items below: without white rice (get brown rice if available) and breadstick. ask for one of the sides above as a replacement*

- Shrimp Skewers
- Blackened Tilapia
- Wild Alaskan Salmon
- Grilled White Fish and Shrimp Skewer
- Lemon Pepper White Fish

# Captain D's Seafood Kitchen (2)

Drink: Water

<u>What's New</u>

- Tilapia & Shrimp Skewer
  *without: white rice (get brown rice if available) and breadstick. instead, ask for one of the sides above as a replacement*
- Lemon Pepper Steamed Shrimp
  *without ketchup or dressing*

# Carl's Jr.

Drink: Water

<u>Sandwiches</u>

- Low Carb Charbroiled Chicken Club
  *without: honey wheat bun (lettuce bun instead), bacon, cheese, and mayo*

<u>Salads</u>

*instead of dressing, ask for: lemon, pepper, vinegar, guacamole/avocados, or fresh salsa*

- Charbroiled Chicken Salad
  *without: cheese, croutons, and dressing*
- Side Salad
  *without: cheese, croutons, and dressing*

# Carraba's Italian Grill

Drink: Water

## Soups

- Minestrone

## Salads

*instead of dressing, ask for: lemon, pepper, vinegar, guacamole/avocados, or fresh salsa*

- Italian Salad
  *without vinaigrette/dressing*
- Johnny Rocco Salad
  *without: vinaigrette/dressing and ricotta*
- Italian Side Salad
  *without vinaigrette/dressing*
- House Side Salad
  *without vinaigrette/dressing*

## Main Plates

*order any of the following without butter or sauce*
*ask for minimal olive oil*

- Tuscan-Grilled Sirloin
- Tuscan-Grilled Filet
- Tuscan-Grilled Ribeye
- Tuscan-Grilled Chicken

## Seafood

- Tomato Basil Salmon
  *ask to be cooked without butter and with little to no oil*
- Wood-Grilled Tilapia
  *without: balsamic glaze. ask for minimal olive oil*
- California Veggie
  *without: cheese*

# Carraba's Italian Grill (2)

Drink: Water

Pasta

- If a whole wheat/grain pasta is available, get it with marinara sauce and meatballs
  *without cheese*

Sides

- Grilled Asparagus
  *without cheese*
- Broccoli
  *ask for broccoli to be grilled or steamed and cooked with little to no oil*

Remember:

**Be brave.**

Do not be afraid to ask waiters to modify menu options! You are paying for the food which directly affects how healthy you look and feel. Be brave and ask for the food you need to succeed.

# Chick-fil-A

Drink: Water

## Breakfast

- Egg White Grill
  *without cheese*
- Sunflower Multigrain Bagel

## Salads

*instead of dressing, ask for: lemon, pepper, vinegar, guacamole/avocados, or fresh salsa*

- Spicy Southwest Salad
  *without: cheese, tortilla strips, and dressing*
- Market Salad
  *without: cheese and dressing*

## Entrées

- Grilled Chicken Cool Wrap
  *without cheese*
- Grilled Chicken Sandwich
  *without sauce*
- Grilled Nuggets
  *without sauce*

## Sides

- Chicken Noodle Soup
  *without saltine crackers*
- Side Salad
  *without cheese*
- Superfood Side
  *without: vinaigrette/dressing, dried sour cherries, and roasted nuts (if sweetened. if plain, they're ok to eat)*
- Fruit Cup

# Chili's Grill & Bar

Drink: Water

## Sides

- Steamed Broccoli
- Black Beans
  *without cheese*
- Corn
  *without butter*
- Grilled Asparagus
  *without butter*

## Salads

*instead of dressing, ask for: lemon, pepper, vinegar, guacamole/avocados, or fresh salsa*

- Santa Fe Chicken Salad
  *without vinaigrette/dressing*
- Quesadilla Explosion Salad
  *without: ricotta and vinaigrette/dressing*
- Grilled Chicken Salad
  *without vinaigrette/dressing*
- Caribbean Salad with Seared Shrimp or Grilled Chicken
  *without vinaigrette/dressing*

## Tacos

- Grilled Chicken or Steak Tacos
  *with: soft corn tortillas, avocado, pico, and cilantro*
  *without: flour tortillas, cheese, coleslaw, and Mexican rice (instead, ask for steamed broccoli, side salad without dressing, cheese, and croutons, or more beans without cheese)*

# Chili's Grill & Bar (2)

Drink: Water

## Guiltless Grill

- Margarita Grilled Chicken
  *without: tortilla strips and Mexican rice (instead, ask for steamed broccoli, side salad without dressing, cheese, and croutons, or beans without cheese)*
- Grilled Chicken Salad
  *without: cheese and vinaigrette/dressing*
- Ancho Salmon
  *without: sauce and cheese. more broccoli instead of white rice (or get brown rice, if available)*
- 6 oz. Classic Sirloin with Grilled Avocado
  *without sauce. and the salad without cheese and dressing*

## Lunch Specials

- Bacon Avocado Grilled Chicken Sandwich
  *without: white bread (whole wheat/grain bread instead), bacon, cheese, sautéed onions (grilled or raw onions instead), mayo, butter, and fries (instead, ask for steamed broccoli, side salad without dressing, cheese, and croutons, or beans without cheese)*
- California Turkey Club
  *without: white bread (whole wheat/grain bread instead), bacon, cheese, sautéed onions (grilled or raw onions instead), mayo, and fries (instead, ask for steamed broccoli, side salad without dressing, cheese, and croutons, or beans without cheese)*
- Chipotle Chicken Fresh Mex Bowl
  *without: cheese, tortilla strips, dressing/sauce (salsa is okay), and Mexican rice (instead, ask for steamed broccoli, side salad without dressing, cheese, and croutons, or beans without cheese)*

# Chili's Grill & Bar (3)

Drink: Water

<u>Fajitas</u>

*ask for fajitas to be cooked with little to no oil*

- Chicken Fajitas
  *without Mexican rice. instead, ask for steamed broccoli, side salad without dressing (lemon instead), cheese, and croutons, or more beans without cheese*
- Steak Fajitas
  *without Mexican rice. instead, ask for steamed broccoli, side salad without dressing (lemon instead), cheese, and croutons, or more beans without cheese*
- Black Bean & Veggie Fajitas
  *without Mexican rice. instead, ask for steamed broccoli, side salad without dressing (lemon instead), cheese, and croutons, or more beans without cheese*

Remember:

**Be consistent.**

Do not take days off. Of course, at first it may be difficult to give up certain things like white bread, dressing, cheese, sugary foods, and butter. Ease off these foods, and notice how your taste buds improve and how great you look and feel.

# Chipotle Mexican Grill

Drink: Water

## Bowl

- Steak
  *with: brown rice, black beans, fresh tomato salsa (mild), roasted chili-corn salsa (medium), lettuce, guacamole (guacamole is extra charge)*
- Chicken
  *with: brown rice, black beans, fresh tomato salsa (mild), roasted chili-corn salsa (medium), lettuce, guacamole (guacamole is extra charge)*
- Barbacoa
  *with: brown rice, black beans, fresh tomato salsa (mild), roasted chili-corn salsa (medium), lettuce, guacamole (guacamole is extra charge)*

## Salad

*instead of dressing, ask for: lemon, pepper, vinegar, guacamole/avocados, or fresh salsa*

- Steak
  *with: brown rice, black beans, fresh tomato salsa (mild), roasted chili-corn salsa (medium), lettuce, guacamole (guacamole is extra charge)*
- Chicken
- *with: brown rice, black beans, fresh tomato salsa (mild), roasted chili-corn salsa (medium), lettuce, guacamole (guacamole is extra charge)*
- Barbacoa
  *with: brown rice, black beans, fresh tomato salsa (mild), roasted chili-corn salsa (medium), lettuce, guacamole (guacamole is extra charge)*

# Chuck E. Cheese's

Drink: Water

## Wraps and Sandwiches

- Club Wrap
  *without: white flour tortilla (whole wheat tortilla instead), bacon, cheese, and mayo*

## Endless Salad Bar

*instead of dressing, ask for: lemon, pepper, vinegar, guacamole/avocados, or fresh salsa*

- Garden-Fresh Salad Bar
  *get any vegetables you want*
  *without: cheese, dressing, and pasta salad*

## Start Your Party Right

- Veggie Platter
  *without dressing*

Remember:

**Think results and after-effects... to say no to junk food now.**

When resisting the temptation to eat unhealthy food, think about how unhealthy junk food makes you feel after you eat it. The healthier you eat, the more you will be able to notice how badly junk food makes the body feel.

# Chuy's

Drink: Water

## Appetizers

- Guacamole
  *without: chips. ask for soft corn tortillas instead*

## Salads & Soups

*instead of dressing, ask for: lemon, pepper, vinegar, guacamole/avocados, or fresh salsa*

- Grilled Chicken Salad
  *without: cheese or dressing*
- Tortilla Soup
  *without cheese and tortilla strips. instead of tortilla strips (usually fried), ask for soft corn tortillas*

## Tacos

- Soft Tacos (Chicken or Beef)
  *ask for soft corn tortillas instead of flour tortillas*
  *without cheese*
- Tacos Al Carbon (Chicken or Beef)
  *ask for soft corn tortillas instead of flour tortillas*
  *without cheese*

## Fajitas

*ask for fajitas to be cooked with little to no oil*

- Chicken Fajitas
  *without: cheese, sour cream, rice, and flour tortillas. ask for more beans or vegetables instead of rice. ask for soft corn tortillas instead of flour tortillas*
- Steak Fajitas
  *without: cheese, sour cream, rice, and flour tortillas. ask for more beans or vegetables instead of rice. ask for soft corn tortillas instead of flour tortillas*

# Cheddar's Scratch Kitchen

Drink: Water

## Soups

- Homemade Baked Potato Soup
  *without: cheese and bacon*
- Tortilla Soup
  *without cheese. instead of tortilla strips (usually fried), ask for soft corn tortillas*

## Salads

*instead of dressing, ask for: lemon, pepper, vinegar, guacamole/avocados, or fresh salsa*

- Grilled Chicken Pecan Salad
  *without: cheese and dressing*
- Salmon & Strawberry Salad
  *without: cheese and dressing*

## Sides

- Steamed Fresh Broccoli
- Baked Potato
  *without: cream, cheese, butter, bacon etc.*
  *optional: pepper, chives*

## Fish

- Grilled Salmon
  *without: cheese and dressing*
- Grilled White Fish
  *without: cheese and dressing*

## Steak

*see above for sides*

- 6 or 8 oz. Top Sirloin Steak
- 12 oz. Ribeye
- 20 oz. Bone-In Ribeye

# Cheddar's Scratch Kitchen (2)

Drink: Water

Lighter Side

- Lemon Pepper White Fish
  *without: salad dressing and white rice (brown rice instead). if brown rice is not available, ask for more beans or salad/vegetables (without dressing, cheese, and croutons) as a substitute*
- Grilled Baja Chicken
  *without white rice (brown rice instead). if not available, ask for more beans without cheese or salad/vegetables (without dressing, cheese, and croutons) as a substitute*

# Cicis Pizza

Drink: Water

Soups & Mini Salads

- Salad Mix
  *without: cheese and dressing*
  *with (optional): grape tomatoes, grape tomatoes, baby carrots, sliced radish, green bell peppers, sliced cucumbers, black olives, broccoli florets, sliced red onions, sliced mushrooms, pineapple, jalapeños, banana peppers*

# Corner Bakery Cafe

Drink: Water

## Featured Flavors

- Farmers Scrambler
  *without: cheese and white bread (get whole wheat/grain toast)*
- Chilled Swiss Oats
  *without: raisin pecan sweet crisp*

## Morning Favorites

- Anaheim Scrambler
  *without: bacon, cheese, and white bread (get whole wheat/grain toast)*

## Oatmeals & Yogurt

- Steel-Cut Oatmeal
  *without: brown sugar and sweet crisp*
- Berry Almond Swiss Oats
  *without sweet crisp*

## Fresh Salads

*instead of dressing, ask for: lemon, pepper, vinegar, guacamole/avocados, or fresh salsa*

- Santa Fe Ranch
  *without: cheese, tortilla strips, and ranch*
- Chopped Salad
  *without: bacon, cheese, and dressing/vinaigrette*
- Harvest Salad
  *without: cheese, pecan sweet crisps, and dressing/vinaigrette*

## Signature Sandwiches

- D.C. Chicken Salad
  *without mayo*
- Uptown Turkey Avocado
  *without: bacon and mayo*

# Corner Bakery Cafe (2)

Drink: Water

Soups

- Roasted Tomato Basil Soup

Power Flats

- Avocado and Spinach
  *without cheese*

Keys to Remember

1. Small changes make a huge difference.
2. Be brave.
3. Be consistent.
4. Think results and after-effects… to say no to junk food now.

# Cracker Barrel Old Country Store

Drink: Water

<u>Breakfast</u>

- Good Morning Breakfast
  *without: turkey sausage and grits. ask for more fruit or eggs instead*
- Custom: ask for scrambled eggs with fruit on the side

<u>Lunch & Dinner</u>

- Southern Chicken Salad
  *without: dressing, Parmesan cheese, croutons, deviled eggs, and dressing. ask for hard-boiled eggs instead*
- Lemon Pepper Grilled Rainbow Trout Plate
  *with sides: fruit, steamed broccoli, carrots, or plain corn*
- Grilled Chicken Salad
  *without: dressing, cheese, croutons, deviled eggs, crackers, and dressing. ask for hard-boiled eggs instead of deviled eggs*
- Grilled Sirloin Steak
  *with: house salad (no dressing, cheese, or croutons) or steamed vegetables*
- 10 oz. Rib Eye Steak
  *without: biscuits and muffins. side: house salad (no dressing, cheese, or croutons), steamed vegetables, or a plain baked potato (no cheese, sour cream, butter, bacon, etc.) optional: pepper, chives*

# Culver's

Drink: Water

Entrées

- Grilled Chicken Sandwich
  *without: white bread (whole wheat/grain or lettuce bun instead)*
- Garden Fresco with Grilled Chicken Salad
  *without: dressing, cheese, and croutons*
- Chicken Cashew With Grilled Chicken
  *without: dressing, cheese, and croutons*
- Vegetable Beef Soup
- Chicken Noodle Soup
  *without noodles*

# Dairy Queen

Drink: Water

Sandwiches

- Grilled Chicken Sandwich
  *without: white bread bun (whole wheat/grain or lettuce bun instead) and mayo*

Salads

- Chicken BLT (Grilled Chicken)
- *without: dressing, bacon, and cheese*
- Side Salad
  *without dressing*

Sides

- Banana

# Dave and Buster's

Drink: Water

Starter Salads & Soups

- Fresh Garden Salad
  *without: cheese, tortilla strips, and dressing*
- Southwestern Tortilla Soup
  *without: cheese and tortilla strips*

Salads

*instead of dressing, ask for: lemon, pepper, vinegar, guacamole/avocados, or fresh salsa*

- Grilled Chicken & Baby Kale
  *without: dressing, cheese, and Parmesan crisp*
- Grilled Steak Salad
  *without: dressing, cheese, candied pecans, and frazzled onions*

Handhelds

- California Smoked Turkey Melt
  *without: white bread (instead, whole wheat/grain bread or a lettuce bun), caramelized onions, cheese, and aïoli*

Remember:

**Small changes make a huge difference.**

Know that the small changes you make add up to make an amazing body through a realistic and physically painless process. Our small choices add up for the better!

# Del Taco

Drink: Water

<u>Handcrafted Salads</u>

- Mexican Chopped Chicken Salad
  *without: cheese, tortilla strips, and dressing*

<u>Street Tacos</u>

*with soft corn tortillas*

- Carne Asada
  *without roasted chile salsa*
- Chicken
  *without roasted chile salsa*

<u>Fresca Bowls</u>

- Pollo Asado With Avocado
  *without white rice (ask for lettuce instead)*
- Avocado Veggie
  *without white rice (ask for lettuce instead)*

Remember:
*The Ocinator Restaurant Diet* is intended to help readers lose body fat, and the Ocinator Fitness Program is intended to help users sculpt abs and other muscles.

# Denny's

Drink: Water

## Fit Fare

- Fit Slam
  *without: turkey bacon and English muffin (unless the English muffin is whole wheat/grain). instead, ask for whole wheat/grain toast or more fruit*
- Loaded Veggie Omelette
  *without: cheese and English muffin (unless the English muffin is whole wheat/grain). instead, ask for whole wheat/grain toast or more fruit*
- Tilapia Ranchero
  *without butter on the corn*
- Veggie Skillet
  *ask for potatoes to be cooked with little to no oil*
- Sirloin Steak
  *without mashed potatoes. instead, ask for whole wheat toast or more vegetables*

## Soups

- Vegetable Beef Soup

## Sandwiches & Salads

*instead of dressing, ask for: lemon, pepper, vinegar, guacamole/avocados, or fresh salsa*

- House Salad
  *without: cheese, croutons, and dressing*
- Tuscan Grilled Chicken Sandwich
- *without: white bread (whole wheat bun instead), bacon, cheese, and mayo*
- Avocado Chicken Caesar Salad
  *without: bacon, cheese, and dressing*

# Denny's (2)

Drink: Water

55+

- 55+ Club Sandwich
  *without: cheese, bacon, mayo, and fries*
  *ask for fruit or steamed vegetables instead of fries*
- 55+ Grilled Tilapia
  *with sides: steamed vegetables, whole wheat/grain toast, or fruit*
- 55+ Grilled Chicken
  *with sides: steamed vegetables, whole wheat/grain toast, or fruit*

Classics & Steaks

- Mediterranean Grilled Chicken
  *with sides: steamed vegetables, whole wheat/grain toast, or fruit*
- Wild Alaska Salmon
  *with sides of steamed vegetables, whole wheat/grain toast, or fruit*
- T-Bone Steak
  *with sides: steamed vegetables, whole wheat/grain toast, or fruit*

# Dickey's Barbecue Pit

Drink: Water

Meat Plates

- Sliced Beef Brisket, Chopped Beef Brisket, Chicken Breast, or Turkey
  *sides: salad without dressing, cheese, and croutons*
  *without: white bread roll and sauce. get more salad instead*

# Domino's

Drink: Water

Salads

*instead of dressing, ask for: lemon, pepper, vinegar, guacamole/avocados, or fresh salsa*

- Classic Garden
  *without: cheese and dressing*
- Chicken Apple Pecan
  *without: cheese and dressing*

# Einstein Bros Bagels

Drink: Water

Classic

- Ancient Grain (Plain)
  *without cream cheese, butter, jam, etc.*

Bread Specialty

- Multigrain Roll (Plain)
  *without cream cheese, butter, jam, etc.*

Remember:
**Stay away from refined grains.**
The prominent advice in medicine today indicates how to lose weight healthily: stay away from products with *refined grain* and products with added sugar. Also, eat lots of vegetables. The key: *refined grain* carbs are bad. On the other hand, *whole grain* carbs are good.

# El Pollo Loco

Drink: Water

Tacos

- Chicken Taco Al Carbon
- Chicken Avocado Taco
  *without: cheese and dressing*

Salads

- Double Chicken Avocado Salad
  *without: sour cream and dressing*
- Classic Salad
  *without: tortilla strips and dressing*
- Mexican Cobb Salad
  *without: bacon, cheese, tortilla strips, and dressing*

Bowls

- Pollo Bowl
  *without: sour cream and dressing*
- Grande Avocado
  *without: tortilla strips and dressing*
- Double Chicken Bowl
  *without: bacon, cheese, tortilla strips, and dressing*
- Chicken Black Bean Bowl
  *without: bacon, cheese, tortilla strips, and dressing*

Family Meals

- 8, 10, 12, or 16 Piece Meal
  *sides: brown rice, black beans, broccoli, loco side salad (without tortilla strips, cheese, and dressing)*

More Chicken

- Skinless Chicken Breast

# Famous Dave's

Drink: Water

## Salads 'N Soups

*instead of dressing, ask for: lemon, pepper, vinegar, guacamole/avocados, or fresh salsa*

- Chicken Chopped Salad
  *without: cheese, tortilla strips, dressing, and corn bread muffin*
  *ask for whole wheat/grain bread or fruit as a substitute*
- Fresh Garden Side Salad
  *without: cheese, bacon, croutons, and dressing*
  *ask for whole wheat/grain bread or fruit as a substitute*
- Mexican Cobb Salad
  *without: bacon, cheese, tortilla strips, and dressing*

## Pitmaster Favorites

*without corn bread muffin. for your two sides, see below*

- Texas Beef Brisket
- Cedar Plank Salmon
  *not glazed and caramelized. just grilled*
- Country-Roasted Chicken

## Side Dishes

- Fresh Steamed Broccoli
  *sides: brown rice, black beans, broccoli, loco side salad (without tortilla strips, cheese, and dressing)*
- Grilled Pineapple Steaks
  *without: cayenne and sugar*

## Lunch

- Baked Potato
  *without: cheese, bacon, sour cream, and butter.*
  *with (optional): pepper, green onions*

# Firehouse Subs

Drink: Water

## Hot or Cold Specialty Subs

- Hook & Ladder
  *without: white bread (whole wheat/grain bread instead), cheese, mayo, and mustard*
- Firehouse Meatball
  *without: white bread (whole wheat/grain bread instead) and cheese*

## Salads

*instead of dressing, ask for: lemon, pepper, vinegar, guacamole/avocados, or fresh salsa*

- Italian With Grilled Chicken Salad
  *without: salami, cheese, and dressing*
- Firehouse Salad
  *without: cheese and dressing*
- Hook & Ladder Salad
  *without: cheese and dressing*

## Hot or Cold Subs

*without cheese, mayo, mustard, and white bread (whole wheat/grain bread instead)*

- Smoked Turkey Breast
- Grilled Chicken Breast
- Virginia Honey Ham

# First Watch

Drink: Water

## The Healthier Side

- Avocado Toast
- Healthy Turkey
  *without feta*
- Power Wrap
- Steel-Cut Oatmeal
  *without: brown sugar and muffin*
- Sunrise Granola Bowl
  *without powdered sugar*
- Tri-Athlete
  *without: cheese and preserves*

## Omelets & Frittatas

- Inspired Italian Omelet
  *without: sausage and cheese*
- Morning Market Vegetable Omelet
  *without: cheese and preserves*

## From The Griddle

- Multigrain Pancakes (Blueberry, Plain, or Banana Granola Crunch)
  *without: butter, syrup, jam, and preserves*

## Power Bowls

- Pesto Chicken Quinoa Bowl
  *without: pesto and feta*
- Power Breakfast Bowl
  *without: sausage, Parmesan, and olive oil. basted eggs with minimal oil, without butter*

# First Watch (2)

Drink: Water

## Salads

*instead of dressing, ask for: lemon, pepper, vinegar, guacamole/avocados, or fresh salsa*

- Chicken Avocado Chop Salad
  *without: cheese, tortilla chips, and dressing*
- Cobb Salad
  *without: bacon, cheese, and dressing*
- Superfood Kale Salad
  *without: Parmesan cheese and vinaigrette/dressing*
- Sweet Honey Pecan Salad
  *without: bacon, cheese, and honey dressing*

## Sandwiches

*without white bread (whole wheat/grain bread instead)*

- Market Veggie
  *without: basil pesto, mayo, and cheese*
- Monterey Club
  *without: bacon, cheese, and mayo*
- Baja Turkey Burger
  *without: mayo and cheese*
- Veggie Burger
  *without: dijonnaise and cheese*

## Juice

- Kale Tonic Fresh Juice

## Sides

- Whole Grain Artisan Toast
  *without preserves*
- Fresh Fruit
- Hearty Vegetable Soup
- Tomato Basil Soup

# Five Guys Burgers and Fries

Drink: Water

<u>Burgers</u>

- Hamburger
  *without: white bread (lettuce bun instead), mayo, mustard, ketchup, relish, bbq sauce, hot sauce, and a1 sauce*

<u>Sandwiches</u>

- Veggie Sandwich
  *without: white bread (lettuce bun instead), mayo, mustard, ketchup, relish, bbq sauce, hot sauce, and a1 sauce*

<u>General Cuisine Guidelines</u>

American

Stay away from: fried food, cheese, sauce, dressing/ vinaigrette, and white bread/buns (including free appetizers).

Choose grilled and whole wheat options.

# Fleming's Prime Steakhouse & Wine Bar

Drink: Water

Chef Curtis' Table

- Porterhouse Steak
  *without bourbon bacon jam*

Salads

*instead of dressing, ask for: lemon, pepper, vinegar, guacamole/avocados, or fresh salsa*

- Seasonal Salad
  *without vinaigrette/dressing*
- Wedge Salad
  *without: bacon, cheese, and dressing*

Sides

- Baked Potato (Plain)
  *without: cheese, sour cream, butter, bacon, etc.*
- Grilled High Country Asparagus

Signature Steaks

*without butter*

- Filet Mignon
- Prime New York Steak

Beyond Steak

- Double Breast of Chicken
- Barbecue Scottish Salmon Fillet
  *without barbecue glaze*

# Freddy's Frozen Custard and Steakburgers

Drink: Water

Burgers

- Steakburger
  *without: white bread (lettuce bun instead), cheese, mustard, ketchup, fries, chips and sauce*

Sandwiches

- Grilled Chicken Breast Sandwich
  *without: white bread, cheese, mustard, ketchup, fries, chips, and sauce*

Be comfortable asking for:

- Whole grains, brown rice - instead of white/refined carbs*
- Food that is steamed, baked/grilled with no/minimal oil
- Lemon slices, vinegar, mustard, guacamole/avocados, or fresh salsa, pepper and other herbs - instead of dressings, condiments and sauces that contain extra oils/fats

*Including free appetizers

# Hardee's

Drink: Water

<u>Sandwiches</u>

- Low Carb Charbroiled Chicken Club
  *without: honey wheat bun (ask for a lettuce bun instead), bacon, cheese, and mayo*

<u>Salads</u>

*instead of dressing, ask for: lemon, pepper, vinegar, guacamole/avocados, or fresh salsa*

- Charbroiled Chicken Salad
  *without: cheese, croutons, and dressing*
- Side Salad
  *without: cheese, croutons, and dressing*

# Hungry Howie's

Drink: Water

<u>Salads</u>

*instead of dressing, ask for: lemon, pepper, vinegar, guacamole/avocados, or fresh salsa*

- Antipasto
  *without: salami, cheese, and dressing*
- Chef
  *without: cheese and dressing*
- Greek
  *without: cheese and dressing*
- Garden
  *without: croutons and dressing*
- Chicken Asiago
  *without: cheese and dressing*
- Chicken Caesar
  *without: cheese and dressing*

# IHOP

Drink: Water or Low-Fat Milk

## Omelettes

*without butter*

- Big Steak Omelette
  *without: cheese and hash browns. with side of fruit or whole wheat/grain toast*
- Chicken Fajita Omelette
  *without: cheese and sour cream. side of fruit or whole wheat/grain toast*
- Spinach & Mushroom Omelette
  *without: cheese and hollandaise. side of fruit or whole wheat/grain toast*
- Egg White Vegetable Omelette
  *without cheese. with side of fruit or whole wheat/grain toast*

## Pancakes

- Harvest Grain 'N Nut
  *without: butter, syrup, jam, preserves, etc. with side of fruit*

## Sandwiches

- Roasted Turkey Sandwich
  *without: bacon, cheese, and mayonnaise*

## Salads

*instead of dressing, ask for: lemon, pepper, vinegar, guacamole/avocados, or fresh salsa*

- Grilled Chicken & Veggie Salad
  *without vinaigrette/dressing*
- Chicken Cobb Salad (Grilled Chicken)
  *without: cheese and dressing*
- House Salad
  *without dressing*

# IHOP (2)

Drink: Water or Low-Fat Milk

Entrées

- Tilapia
  *without: alfredo sauce and mashed potatoes. instead, ask for whole wheat/grain toast or fruit*

# In-N-Out

Drink: Water

Burgers

- Protein-Style Hamburger
  *without: white bread bun (lettuce bun instead), cheese, and sauce without fries*
- Protein-Style Double Meat
  *without: white bread bun (lettuce bun instead), cheese, and sauce without fries*

Remember:

**Stay away from refined grains.**

*Refined grain* carbs are unhealthy because they have been stripped of the nutrients that whole grains have. But because *whole grain* carbs have those nutrients, they are good for you.

# Jamba Juice

Drink: Water

<u>Fruit & Veggie Smoothies</u>

- Apple 'n Greens Smoothie
- Greens 'n Ginger Smoothie
- Berry UpBEET Smoothie
- Apple 'n Greens Smoothie
- Orange Carrot Karma Smoothie

<u>All Fruit Smoothies</u>

- Mega Mango Smoothie
- Peach Perfection Smoothie
- Pomegranate Paradise Smoothie
- Strawberry Whirl Smoothie
- Orange Carrot Karma Smoothie

<u>Bowls</u>

- Peachy Green Goodness Bowl
- Fruit and Greek Yogurt Bowl

<u>Tasty Bites</u>

- Oatmeal

<u>Protein Smoothies</u>

- Fruit and Greek Yogurt Bowl

<u>Boosts</u>

- Greek Yogurt Boost
- Kale Boost
- Chia Seed Boost
- Chia Topper
- Pumpkin Seed Boost

# Jason's Deli

Drink: Water

## Specialty Sandwiches

*instead of dressing, ask for: lemon, pepper, vinegar, guacamole/avocados, or fresh salsa*

- Santa Fe Chicken Sandwich
  *without: white bread (multigrain bread instead), bacon, cheese, and dressing*
- MeataBalla
  *without: French bread (whole wheat/grain bread instead) and cheese*
- Amy's Turkey-O
  *without: white bread (whole wheat/grain bread instead), cheese, and mustard*
- JB's Southwest Turkey
  *without: white bread (whole wheat/grain bread instead), cheese, and aïoli*

## Wraps

- Turkey Wrap
  *without ranch. with side of fruit or steamed veggies*
- Mediterranean Wrap
  *without hummus. with side of fruit or steamed veggies*
- Ranchero Wrap
  *without cheddar jalapeños. with side of fruit or steamed veggies*

## Famous Favorites

- Wild Salmon-wich
  *without: white bread (whole wheat/grain bread instead) and aïoli with side of fruit or steamed veggies*

## Soups

- Organic Vegetable
- Tomato Basil

# Jason's Deli (2)

Drink: Water

## Build Your Own Sandwich

*instead of dressing, ask for: lemon, pepper, vinegar, guacamole/avocados, or fresh salsa*

- Meats
  *Ham, Roasted Turkey Breast, Smoked Turkey Breast, Pineapple*
- Breads
  *Multigrain Wheat, Rye, Gluten-Free Bread, Organic Wheat Wrap, Organic Ancient Grain Bun*
  *without: white bread, white flour tortilla*
- Add-Ons
  *Guacamole, Avocado Slices*
- Spreads and Cheeses
  *without spreads and cheese (vinegar and/or pepper instead)*

## Salads

*instead of dressing, ask for: lemon, pepper, vinegar, guacamole/avocados, or fresh salsa*

- Chicken Club Salad
  *without: bacon, cheese, dressing*
- Nutty Mixed-Up Salad
  *without: cheese and dressing*
- Mesa Chicken Salad
  *without: cheese and dressing*
- Salmon Pacifica Salad
  *without vinaigrette/dressing*
- The Big Chef
  *without cheese*

## Potatoes

- Pollo Mexicano Potato
  *without: cheese, sour cream, and butter*

# Jason's Deli (3)

Drink: Water

Meatless Eats

- Spinach Veggie Wrap
  *without: white flour wrap (whole wheat/grain wrap instead) and cheese*
  *with side of fruit, steamed veggies, or baked chips*
- Fresh Fruit
  *without creamy dip*
- Zucchini Grillini
  *ask for bread to have very little olive oil*
  *without white bread (whole wheat/grain bread instead) and cheese*
  *with side of fruit, steamed veggies, or baked chips*
- Black Bean Taco Salad
  *without: blue corn chips (unless baked), cheese, and sour cream. ask for baked chips, steamed veggies, or fruit instead of blue corn chips*

# Jet's Pizza

Drink: Water

Salads

*instead of dressing, ask for: lemon, pepper, vinegar, guacamole/avocados, or fresh salsa*

- Antipasto Salad
  *without: salami, cheese, and dressing*
- Garden Salad
  *without: cheese and dressing*
- Greek Salad
  *without: cheese and dressing*
- Chicken Caesar Salad
  *without: Parmesan, croutons, and dressing*

# Jersey Mike's Subs

Drink: Water

<u>Cold Subs</u>

*with whole wheat/grain bread (without white bread)*
*without: cheese, mayo, olive oil, and white bread*
*instead of dressing, ask for: lemon, pepper, vinegar, guacamole/avocados, or fresh salsa*

- #3 The American Classic (Ham)
- #14 The Veggie
- #7 Turkey Breast
- #6 Famous Roast Beef
- #8 Cold Sub (Turkey & Ham)

Remember:

**Stay away from products with added sugar and artificial sweeteners.**

Stay away from: soda, most desserts, dressings, syrups, jams, jellies, etc. Instead, try eating naturally sweet food like fruit.

# Jimmy John's Gourmet Sandwiches

Drink: Water

<u>Classics</u>

*with whole wheat/grain bread (without white bread)*
*without: white bread, dijon, cheese, mayo, and olive oil*
*instead of dressing, ask for: lemon, pepper, vinegar, guacamole/avocados, or fresh salsa*

- #2 Original Roast Beef
- #4 Turkey Breast
- #1 Ham
- #6 Veggie

<u>Favorites</u>

*with whole wheat/grain bread (without white bread)*
*without: dijon, cheese, mayo, and white bread*
*instead of dressing, ask for: lemon, pepper, vinegar, guacamole/avocados, or fresh salsa*

- #8 Roast Beef & Ham
- #10 Double Roast Beef
- #14 Roast Beef & Turkey Breast
- #7 Double Ham
- #11 Turkey & Ham
- #13 Veggie Club

# KFC

Drink: Water

Grilled Chicken

- 8, 12, and 16 pc. Bucket Meal
  *without biscuits. ask to substitute side below instead of biscuits*

Sides

- Green Beans
- Corn (if available without butter)

Remember:
**Stay away from refined grains.**
Studies have shown that not eating whole grain carbs could lead to: poorer memory-based task performance, bad breath, and increased anger, depression, anxiety, irritability, and hostility.

# Logan's Roadhouse

- Drink: Water

## Salads & Soups

*instead of dressing, ask for: lemon, pepper, vinegar, guacamole/avocados, or fresh salsa*

- Mesquite Grilled Chicken Salad
  *without: cheese, croutons, and dressing*
- Roadhouse Steak Cobb Salad
  *without: bacon, cheese, croutons, and dressing*
- Fresh Garden Salad
  *without: cheese, croutons, and dressing*

## Sides

- Baked Potato (Plain)
  *without: cheese, sour cream, butter, bacon, etc.*
- Steamed Broccoli
- Fresh Garden Salad
  *without: cheese, croutons, and dressing*
- Roasted Corn Salad (Seasonal Special)
  *without: vinaigrette and cheese*
- Corn
  *without butter*

## Burgers & Sandwiches

*without fries or chips. see sides above for substitutes*

- Logan's Club
  *without: white bread (whole wheat/grain bread or a lettuce bun instead), bacon, cheese, and mayo*
- Grilled Chicken Sandwich
  *without: white bread (whole wheat/grain bread or a lettuce bun instead), bacon, cheese, and mayo*

# Logan's Roadhouse (2)

Drink: Water

<u>Chicken & Seafood</u>

*see sides section above*

- Logan's Wood-Grilled Chicken
  *without: Parmesan peppercorn dressing and white rice. ask for more salad without dressing instead*
- Mesquite Wood-Grilled Salmon
  *without: white rice and sauce. ask for more salad without dressing instead*
- Lemon Herb Chicken
  *without: butter and white rice. ask for more salad without dressing instead*

<u>Steak</u>

- Top Sirloin
  *without mayo*
- Filet Mignon
  *without: white bread, cheese, and olive oil*
- New York Strip
  *without: white bread, cheese, and olive oil*

# Long John Silver's

Drink: Water

<u>Baked Meals</u>

- Baked Cod Meal
  *without: white rice and hushpuppies. ask for steamed vegetables or a salad without dressing, croutons, or cheese instead*

# Longhorn Steakhouse

Drink: Water

## Legendary Steaks

*get double salad (without dressing, cheese, croutons) instead of a side. also, don't eat the steak fat*

- Renegade Sirloin
  *without butter*
- Outlaw Ribeye
  *without butter*
- New York Strip
  *without butter*
- Flat Iron Steak
  *without butter*
- Fire-Grilled T-Bone
  *without butter*
- The Longhorn
  *without butter*

## Salad

*instead of dressing, ask for: lemon, pepper, vinegar, guacamole/avocados, or fresh salsa*

- Grilled Chicken & Strawberry Salad
  *without: candied pecans, feta, and raspberry vinaigrette*
- 7-Pepper Sirloin Salad
  *without: cheese, croutons, and dressing*

## Sides

- Mixed Green Salad
  *without: dressing, croutons, and cheese*
- 7-Pepper Sirloin Salad
  *without: cheese, croutons, and dressing*

# Maggiano's Little Italy

Drink: Water

## Salad

*instead of dressing, ask for: lemon, pepper, vinegar, guacamole/avocados, or fresh salsa*

- Italian Tossed Salad
  *without: pepperoncini, croutons, and vinaigrette/dressing*
- Grilled Salmon Salad
  *without: croutons and vinaigrette/dressing*
- Grilled Chicken Salad
  *without: mozzarella, croutons, and vinaigrette/dressing*

## Sides

- Fresh Grilled Asparagus
  *without: cheese, croutons, and vinaigrette/dressing*

## On The House Classic Pastas

*get whole wheat penne, or gluten-free if you have gluten sensitivities*

- Whole Wheat Penne with Marinara
- Whole Wheat Penne with Meatball
- Whole Wheat Penne with Meat Sauce

## Seafood

- Grilled Salmon Lemon & Herb
  *without white wine butter sauce*

## Chicken

- Grilled Chicken (a la carte)

# Maggiano's Little Italy (2)

Drink: Water

Steak & Veal

- Filet Mignon
  *without asparagus risotto. ask for grilled or steamed asparagus instead*
- Center-Cut Filet Mignon
  *without: garlic butter and crispy vesuvio potatoes. ask for steamed or grilled potatoes instead*

# Marco's Pizza

Drink: Water

Salads

*instead of dressing, ask for: lemon, pepper, vinegar, guacamole/avocados, or fresh salsa*

- Antipasto
  *without: salami, cheese, and dressing*
- Chicken Caesar
  *without: Parmesan cheese, croutons, and dressing*
- Greek
  *without: feta cheese and dressing*
- Garden
  *without: cheddar cheese, croutons, and dressing*

# McAlister's Deli

Drink: Water

## Sandwiches

*with whole wheat/grain bread and wraps*
*without white bread or white flour wraps*
*instead of dressing, ask for: lemon, pepper, vinegar, guacamole/avocados, or fresh salsa*

- The McAlister's Club
  *without: white bread, bacon, cheddar, Swiss, mayo, and mustard*
- King Club
  *without: white bread, bacon, cheddar, Swiss, mayo, and mustard*
- McAlister's Club Wrap
  *without: white flour wrap, bacon, cheddar, Swiss, mayo, and mustard*
- Black Angus Club
  *without: white bread, bacon, cheddar, Swiss, mayo, and horseradish sauce*
- Grilled Chicken Club
  *without: white bread, bacon, cheddar, Swiss, mayo, and honey mustard sauce*
- Turkey Cobb
  *without: white bread, bacon, cheese, mayo, and ranch*
- Garden Fresh Turkey
  *without: white bread, cheese, and vinaigrette*
- The Veggie
  *without: white bread and mayo*

## Soups

- Fire Roasted Vegetable
- Chicken Tortilla
  *without: cheese and tortilla strips*
- Tomato Bisque

# McAlister's Deli (2)

Drink: Water

<u>Salads</u>

*instead of dressing, ask for: lemon, pepper, vinegar, guacamole/avocados, or fresh salsa*

- Savannah Chopped Salad
  *without: honey roasted almonds, gorgonzola, and dressing*
- Southwest Cobb
  *without: cheese, tortilla chips, and dressing*
- Italian Chopped Salad
  *without: salami, cheese, and dressing*
- Grilled Chicken Salad
  *without: cheese, croutons, and dressing*
- Grilled Chicken Salad
  *without: cheese, croutons, and dressing*
- Chef Salad
  *without: bacon, cheese, croutons, and dressing*
- Garden Salad
  *without: cheese, croutons, and dressing*

Remember:
Eating whole grain carbs could lead to positive effects by allowing the soluble fiber, found in whole grain carbs, to:

- Decrease LDL (bad) cholesterol
- Increase good HDL cholesterol
- Increase dietary fiber
- Help promote fat loss
- Prevent fat gain
- Lower the risk of diabetes

# McDonald's

Drink: Water

## Sandwiches

- Artisan Grilled Chicken Sandwich
  *without: white bread (lettuce bun instead) and sauce*

## Salads

*instead of dressing, ask for: lemon, pepper, vinegar, guacamole/avocados, or fresh salsa*

- Bacon and Ranch Grilled Chicken Salad
  *without: bacon, ranch, and cheese*
- Southwest Grilled Chicken Salad
  *without: cheese, tortilla strips, dressing, and cilantro lime glaze*
- Side Salad
  *without dressing*

## Sides

- Kids' Apple Slices

Remember:
**Stay away from products with added sugar and artificial sweeteners.**
The more you stay away from products with added sugar, the sweeter naturally sweet food, like fruit, will taste!

# Mellow Mushroom

Drink: Water

## Salads

*instead of dressing, ask for: lemon, pepper, vinegar, guacamole/avocados, or fresh salsa*

- Greek Salad
  *without feta cheese*
- House Salad
  *without: Parmesan cheese and vinaigrette/dressing*
- Chef Salad
  *without: mozzarella, provolone, and dressing*

## Munchies

- Meatball Trio
  *without: mozzarella, Parmesan, and breadcrumbs*

## Sandwiches & Hoagies

- Chicken Caesar Wrap
  *without: white flour wrap (multigrain wrap instead) and sauce*
- Country Club
  *without: white bread (multigrain bread instead) and sauce*
- California Club
  *without: white bread (multigrain bread instead) and sauce*
- Avocado Hoagie
  *without: white bread (multigrain roll instead), provolone, and mayo*
- Meatball Hoagie
  *without: white bread (multigrain roll instead) and mozzarella*

# Miller's Ale House

Drink: Water

## On The Greens

*instead of dressing, ask for: lemon, pepper, vinegar, guacamole/avocados, or fresh salsa*

- Asian Grilled Chicken Salad
  *without: crispy rice noodles and sesame-ginger vinaigrette*
- Blackened Chicken Breast Salad
  *without: cheese, crispy tortilla strips, garlic-lime crema, and vinaigrette/dressing*
- House Salad
  *without: cheese, croutons, and vinaigrette/dressing*
- Southwest Seared Flat Iron Steak Salad
  *without: cheese, crispy onion tanglers, Dijon-horseradish drizzle, and vinaigrette/dressing*

## Two Hand Grip

- Grilled Chicken Breast Sandwich
  *without brioche bun (lettuce bun instead). with guacamole and fresh pico de gallo*
- Mahi-Mahi Sandwich
  *without: brioche bun (lettuce bun instead) and tartar sauce*

## From The Grill

*with steamed vegetables*

- Center Cut Sirloin
- Flat Iron Steak
- Filet Mignon
- Ribeye

# Miller's Ale House (2)

Drink: Water

From The Sea

*with steamed vegetables*

- Atlantic Salmon
  *without: coleslaw and tartar sauce*
- Mahi-Mahi
  *without: coleslaw and tartar sauce*
- North Atlantic Lobster Tail
  *without butter*

Fajitas

*with grilled (not sautéed) vegetables*
*without cheese, sour cream, flour tortillas*

- Grilled Marinated Chicken Breast
- Grilled Flat Iron Steak
- Steak and Chicken Combo

Sides

- Baked Potato
  *without: butter, sour cream, etc.*
- Seasonal Vegetable
  *steamed or grilled*
- Beans

# Moe's Southwest Grill

Drink: Water

## Burritos

- Homewrecker Mexican Burrito With Guac (Steak, Chicken, Fish, or Tofu)
  *without: white flour tortilla (whole wheat/grain tortilla instead), white rice, cheese, sour cream, ranch, vinaigrette, bacon, and queso*
- Joey Southwest Burrito (Steak, Chicken, Fish, or Tofu)
  *without: white flour tortilla (whole wheat/grain tortilla instead), white rice, cheese, sour cream, ranch, vinaigrette, bacon, and queso*

## Bowls

- Bowl'd Southwest Flavors Earmuffs (Steak, Chicken, Fish, or Tofu)
  *without: white rice, cheese, sour cream, ranch, vinaigrette, bacon, and queso.*

## Tacos

- Steak or Chicken
  *without: avocado lime crema, queso fresco, slaw, sour cream, ranch, vinaigrette, bacon, and queso. with soft corn tortilla*

## Salads

*instead of dressing, ask for: lemon, pepper, vinegar, guacamole/avocados, or fresh salsa*

- Chicken, Steak, Fish, or Tofu
  *without: avocado lime crema, queso fresco, slaw, sour cream, ranch, vinaigrette, bacon, and queso. don't eat the hard shell (fried) bowl*

## Sides

- Pico de Gallo
- Guacamole

# Moe's Southwest Grill (2)

Drink: Water

Stacks

- Steak, Chicken, Fish, or Tofu
  *without: white flour tortilla (whole grain tortilla instead), fried hard corn tortillas (soft corn tortillas instead) white rice, cheese, sour cream, ranch, vinaigrette, bacon, and queso*

Remember:
**Stay away from products with added sugar and artificial sweeteners.**
Look out for hidden sugars and additives. For example, dressing contains too much added sugar, as well as saturated fat and sodium that can lead to increased body fat and feelings of hunger.

# Ninety Nine Restaurant & Pub

Drink: Water

## Burgers

*with steamed vegetables or side salad without dressing*

- West Coast Turkey Burger
  *without: white bread (whole wheat/grain bun/bread or lettuce bun instead) and cheese*
- Vegetarian Black Bean Burger
  *without: white bread (whole wheat/grain bun/bread or lettuce bun instead) and dressing (on salad)*
- Burger
  *without: white bread (whole wheat/grain bun/bread or lettuce bun instead) and cheese*

## Sandwiches

- Triple-Decker Turkey Club
  *without: bacon and cheese*

## 9.99

*see below for sides*

- Grilled Chicken
  *without balsamic glaze*
- Grilled Ribeye Steak
  *without bacon marmalade*
- Chopped Grilled Angus
  *without: mashed potatoes, red wine sauce, sautéed mushrooms, and crispy onions. ask for grilled or steamed vegetables instead*

# Ninety Nine Restaurant & Pub (2)

Drink: Water

## Salads

*instead of dressing, ask for: lemon, pepper, vinegar, guacamole/avocados, or fresh salsa*

- Sundried Tomato Chicken Kabob Salad
  *without: feta cheese, croutons, and dressing*
- Sirloin Tip Heart of Caesar Salad
  *without: Caesar dressing, bacon, croutons, and Parmesan cheese*

## Chicken, Turkey & More

*with steamed vegetables or side salad without dressing*

- Grilled Turkey Tip Skewers
  *without: white bread (whole wheat/grain bun/bread or lettuce instead), sauce, and vinaigrette/dressing*

## Seafood

*see sides section for side choices*

- Fresh Salmon
  *without feta cheese*

## Gluten Sensitive

*see above for duplicates. sides: in-season vegetable (grilled or steamed) or baked potato (plain)*

- Fresh Seasoned Salmon
- Royal Sirloin
  *without cheese and dressing on salad*
- Broiled Sirloin Tips
  *without cheese and dressing on salad*

# Ninety Nine Restaurant & Pub (3)

- Drink: Water

Gluten Sensitive Side Salads

- Heart of Caesar Side Salad
  *without: bacon, croutons, and dressing*
- Garden Side Salad
  *without: Parmesan, croutons, and dressing*

Steaks and Ribs

- Royal Sirloin
  *without cheese and dressing on salad*
- Broiled Sirloin Tips
  *without cheese and dressing on salad*
- Top Sirloin Steak
  *without cheese and dressing on salad*

Remember:
**Stay away from products with added sugar and artificial sweeteners.**
Research changes regarding the side effects of artificial sweeteners, so it is best to avoid them.

# Noodles World Kitchen

Drink: Water

<u>Veggie Noodles</u>

- Zucchini with Grilled Chicken
  *without: sauce, cream, and cheese*
- Zucchini Romesco
  *without: red pepper sauce, cream, and feta*

<u>Salads</u>

*instead of dressing, ask for: lemon, pepper, vinegar, guacamole/avocados, or fresh salsa*

- The Med Salad With Chicken
  *without: spicy yogurt dressing, cavatappi pasta (if possible, ask for zucchini pasta instead), and feta*
- Chicken Veracruz Salad
  *without: chili-lime chicken (grilled chicken instead), bacon, dressing, and crispy jalapeños*
- Grilled Chicken Caesar
  *without: dressing, croutons, and Parmesan*

<u>Soups</u>

- Tomato Basil Bisque
- Chicken Noodle Soup
  *without noodles (or with plain zucchini noodles, if possible)*

<u>Sides</u>

- Tomato Basil Bisque
- Chicken Noodle Soup
  *without noodles*
- Tossed Green Side Salad
  *without: vinaigrette/dressing*
- Caesar Side Salad
  *without: dressing, croutons, and Parmesan*

# O'Charley's

Drink: Water

<u>Soups, Salads, and Sides</u>

*instead of dressing, ask for: lemon, pepper, vinegar, guacamole/avocados, or fresh salsa*

- Southern Pecan Chicken Tender Salad
  *without: dried cranberries, cheese, candied pecans, and dressing/vinaigrette*
- Sonoma Chicken Salad
  *without: dressing and bbq sauce*
- California Chicken Salad
  *without: cheese, candied pecans, dried cranberries, and dressing/vinaigrette*
- The Classic Cobb
  *without: cheese, bacon, croutons, and dressing/vinaigrette*
- Steakhouse Wedge Salad
  *without: cheese and dressing/vinaigrette*
- Chicken Tortilla Soup
  *without: cheese and tortilla strips*
- Chicken Harvest Soup
  *without: cheese*
- Fresh Broccoli
- Baked Potato (Plain)
  *without: butter, sour cream, cheese, bacon, etc.*
- Fresh Grilled Asparagus

<u>Over The Top And Under $10</u>

- Chopped Steak
  *without gravy, fried onions, and bacon smashed potatoes. ask for sides from above instead*
- Santa Fe Tilapia
  *without white rice. ask for a side from above instead*

# O'Charley's (2)

Drink: Water

## Sunday Brunch

*without white bread toast (whole wheat/grain bread instead)*

- Veggie Omelet
  *without: cheese, butter, and Parmesan potatoes (ask for more fruit or toast instead)*
- Country Scramble
  *without: cheese, butter, sausage, bacon, and Parmesan potatoes (ask for more fruit or toast instead)*
- Ultimate Omelette
  *without: cheese, butter, and Parmesan potatoes (ask for a side from above instead)*

## Fresh Burgers & Sandwiches

*instead of fries: fresh broccoli, baked potato, fresh grilled asparagus, or fruit*

- The Club Sandwich
  *without: white bread (whole wheat/grain bread instead), bacon, cheese, mayo, and honey mustard*

## Steaks, Ribs, & Prime Rib

*sides: fresh broccoli, baked potato, fresh grilled asparagus, or fruit*

- Grilled Top Sirloin
- Filet Mignon
  *without garlic butter*

## Seafood Favorites

*sides: fresh broccoli, baked potato, fresh grilled asparagus, or fruit*

- Fresh Cedar-Planked Salmon
- Fresh Grilled Atlantic Salmon

## Classic Combos

*sides: fresh broccoli, baked potato, fresh grilled asparagus, or fruit*

- Steak & Grilled Atlantic Salmon

# Olive Garden

Drink: Water

Note: don't eat breadsticks (made with white bread)

## Soups & Salads

*instead of dressing, ask for: lemon, pepper, vinegar, guacamole/avocados, or fresh salsa*

- ToGo Our Famous House Salad
  *without: cheese, dressing, and croutons*
- Minestrone
- Unlimited Our Famous House Salad
  *without: cheese, dressing, and croutons*

## Cucina Mia! – Create Your Own Pasta Bowl

- Whole Grain Linguine
  *with: traditional marinara or traditional meat sauce; meatballs, grilled chicken, or garden veggies*
- Gluten-Free Rotini
  *with: traditional marinara or traditional meat sauce; meatballs, grilled chicken, or garden veggies*

## Tastes Of The Mediterranean

- Salmon Piccata
  *without: garlic butter sauce and Parmesan-crusted zucchini (ask for grilled vegetables instead)*
- Herb-Grilled Salmon
  *without: garlic butter sauce and Parmesan-crusted zucchini (ask for grilled vegetables instead)*

# Olive Garden (2)

- Drink: Water

<u>Chicken</u>

- Chicken Giardino
  *with: whole wheat pasta instead of pappardelle pasta. or gluten-free pasta if you have gluten sensitivities*
  *without: bacon, cheese, mayo, honey mustard, and white bread (ask for grilled vegetables instead)*
- Chicken Piccata
  *without: garlic butter sauce and Parmesan-crusted zucchini (ask for grilled vegetables instead)*

<u>Beef</u>

- 6 oz Sirloin
  *without: garlic butter, Parmesan-crusted zucchini (ask for grilled vegetables instead), fettuccine alfredo (instead, whole wheat pasta, or gluten-free pasta if you have gluten sensitivities, and marinara or meat sauce)*

Remember:
**Stay away from products with added sugar and artificial sweeteners.**
Small changes like eating fruit and getting rid of salad dressing add up and make a huge difference!

# On The Border

Drink: Water

## Starters

- Guacamole

## Soup & Salads

*instead of dressing, ask for: lemon, pepper, vinegar, guacamole/avocados, or fresh salsa*

- Chicken Tortilla Soup
  *without: cheese and tortilla strips*
- Grande Taco Salad
  *without: cheese, sour cream sauce, flour tortilla crisps, and dressing*
- Fajita Salad
  *ask for fajitas to be cooked with little to no oil*
  *without queso fresco and dressing*
- Mango Chicken Salad
  *without: queso fresco, vinaigrette, and dressing*

## Tacos

- Southwest Chicken Tacos
  *without: flour tortillas (soft corn tortillas instead), cheese, creamy red chile sauce, and fried onion strings*
- Street-Style Mini Tacos (Steak or Chicken)
  *without: sautéed onion and cheese*
- Grilled Fish Tacos Del Mar
  *without: chimichurri, lime cabbage-carrot slaw, and mayo*

## Fajitas

*with soft corn tortillas instead of flour tortillas, beans, pico de gallo, and guacamole. without rice (extra of one of the options above instead)*

- Classic Fajitas (Chicken, Steak, or Portobello & Vegetables)
  *ask for fajitas to be cooked with little to no oil*

# On The Border (2)

Drink: Water

## Favorites

*instead of rice, ask for grilled vegetables or beans without cheese*

- Grilled Fiesta Chicken
  *without: queso, sautéed vegetables, and rice*
- Mexican Grilled Chicken
  *without rice*
- Carne Asada
  *without rice*

## Border Bowls

- Border Bowls (Chicken or Steak without chimichurri)
  *without: rice and queso*

## Sides

- Black Beans
  *without cheese*
- Refried Beans
  *without cheese*
- Corn Tortillas
- Guacamole
- Avocado Slices
- Taco (Chicken Tinga or Beef)
  *with soft corn tortilla*
  *without: white flour tortilla and cheese*

## Party Platters

- Tacos (Chicken Tinga or Beef)
  *with soft corn tortillas*
  *without cheese*

# On The Border (3)

Drink: Water

Family Meals

- Fajita Family Meal (Chicken or Steak)
  *without: flour tortillas (get soft corn tortillas instead), sour cream, and cheese. ask for fajitas to be cooked with little to no oil*
- Taco Family Meal (Chicken Tinga or Beef)
  *with soft corn tortillas*
  *without cheese*

Remember:

**Balance your meats.**

Though this book lists beef menu options, it is not a free pass to eat beef during every meal. Try eating mostly chicken and fish. Consuming too much red meat can be unhealthy.

# Outback Steakhouse

Drink: Water

## Starters

- Guacamole

## Soups & Side Salads

*instead of dressing, ask for: lemon, pepper, vinegar, guacamole/avocados, or fresh salsa*

- Chicken Tortilla Soup
  *without: cheese and tortilla strips*
- House Salad
  *without: dressing, cheese, and croutons*

## Lunch Sides

- Baked Potato (Plain)
  *without: butter, cheese, sour cream, bacon, etc.*
- Sweet Potato (Plain)
  *without: honey butter and brown sugar*
- Grilled Asparagus
  *without olive oil*

## Signature Steaks

*with plain baked potato, salad, and side from above*

- Outback Center-Cut Sirloin
- Victoria's Filet Mignon
  *without: queso, sautéed vegetables, and white rice (ask for grilled vegetables or beans without cheese instead)*
- Ribeye

# Outback Steakhouse (2)

Drink: Water

<u>Chicken, Ribs, Chops & More</u>

- Grilled Chicken On The Barbie
  *without bbq sauce*
- Perfectly Grilled Salmon
  *without bbq sauce*
- Simply Grilled Tilapia
  *without bbq sauce*

<u>Steak And Lobster</u>

- Victoria's Filet Mignon & Lobster
  *without butter*
- Bone-In Natural Cut Ribeye
  *without: butter, cheese, sour cream, and bacon on potato*

<u>Walkabout Wednesday</u>

*without fries. instead: plain baked potato, salad, or side from above (they might charge extra)*

- 6 Oz Center-Cut Sirloin
- Grilled Chicken On The Barbie

<u>Steak Mates</u>

- Steamed Lobster Tail
  *without butter*
- Perfectly Grilled Salmon
- *without bbq sauce*
- Simply Grilled Tilapia
  *without bbq sauce*

# Panda Express

Drink: Water

Sides

- Mixed Vegetables
- Brown Steamed Rice

# Panera Bread

Drink: Water

Soups

- Low-Fat Chicken Noodle Soup
- Black Bean Soup

Salads

*instead of dressing, ask for: lemon, pepper, vinegar, guacamole/avocados, or fresh salsa*

- Strawberry Poppyseed Salad With Chicken
  *without: dressing and oil roasted pecans*
- Asian Sesame Salad with Chicken
  *without: Asian sesame vinaigrette and wonton strips*
- Southwest Chile Lime Ranch Salad with Chicken
  *without: masa chips, dressing, and feta*
- Modern Greek Salad with Quinoa
  *without: dressing and feta*
- Green Goddess Cobb Salad with Chicken
  *without: pickled onions, dressing, mayonnaise, and bacon*
- Fuji Apple Salad with Chicken
  *without: dressing, apple chips, oil roasted pecans, and Gorgonzola*
- Greek Salad
  *without: feta and dressing*
- Caesar Salad with Chicken
  *without: Parmesan, croutons, and dressing*
- Seasonal Greens Salad
  *without vinaigrette/dressing*

# Panera Bread (2)

Drink: Water

<u>Sandwiches</u>

- Turkey Sandwich (whole or half)
  *without: mayo and mustard*
- Ham Sandwich
  *without: Swiss, mayo, and mustard*
- Mediterranean Veggie Sandwich
  *without: tomato basil bread (whole wheat/grain bread instead), feta, and hummus*
- Roasted Turkey & Avocado BLT
  *without white bread (whole wheat/grain bread instead), bacon, and mayo*

<u>Breakfast Sandwiches</u>

- Avocado, Egg White & Spinach
  *without: bagel (ask for whole wheat/grain bread instead) and cheddar*
- Ham & Egg
  *without cheese*

<u>Freshly Baked Breads</u>

- Rye
- Whole Grain

# Papa John's

Drink: Water

<u>Papa's Salads</u>

*instead of dressing, ask for: lemon, pepper, vinegar, guacamole/avocados, or fresh salsa*

- Papa's Garden Salad
  *without: dressing, croutons, and cheese*
- Chicken Caesar Salad
  *without: cheese, croutons, and Caesar dressing*

# Pappadeaux Seafood Kitchen

Drink: Water

## Soups & Salads

*instead of dressing, ask for: lemon, pepper, vinegar, guacamole/avocados, or fresh salsa*

- Pappas Greek Salad
  *without: feta cheese and dressing*
- Pappadeaux House Salad
  *without: croutons, bacon, cheddar, and dressing*
- Classic Caesar
  *without: croutons, Parmesan cheese, and Caesar dressing*
- Chopped Salad (with Grilled Salmon)
  *without: bacon, cheese, vinaigrette, fried chicken, and fried crawfish*
- Seafood Cobb Salad
  *without: bacon, cheese, and vinaigrette/dressing*

## Chef Selections

- Rainbow Trout & Shrimp
  *without: butter sauce and sautéed spinach (ask for grilled spinach or other vegetable instead)*
- Halibut & Spanish Octopus
  *without butter sauce*
- Grilled Tilapia & Jumbo Shrimp
  *without butter*
- Grilled Redfish & Jumbo Shrimp
  *without: butter and risotto*
- Atlantic Salmon Yvette
  *without: white wine sauce and white rice (ask for grilled vegetables or a salad without dressing, cheese, and croutons instead)*

# Pappadeaux Seafood Kitchen (2)

Drink: Water

Steak, Lobster & Crab

- Prime Beef Rib-Eye
  *without: mashed potatoes (and ask for broccolini to be steamed or grilled, not sautéed)*
- Filet Mignon
  *without: butter and mashed potatoes (and ask for asparagus to be steamed or grilled, not sautéed)*
- Filet Mignon & Grilled Rock Lobster
  *without: butter and mashed potatoes*
- Grilled Caribbean Lobster Tail
  *without: butter and mashed potatoes (and ask for broccolini to be steamed or grilled, not sautéed)*

Remember:
**Eat lots of vegetables.**
We all know the many benefits of eating most vegetables! Fiber and vitamins and minerals help us look and feel fresh.

# Pei Wei Asian Diner

Drink: Water

<u>Small Plates, Shareables & Soups</u>

- Edamame
  *without: feta cheese and dressing*

<u>Chef Selections</u>

*instead of dressing, ask for: lemon, pepper, vinegar, guacamole/avocados, or fresh salsa*

- Kale Quinoa Chicken Salad
  *without: tangy Asian slaw, vinaigrette, and dressing*
- Ahi Avocado Salad
  *without: Asian slaw, pickled ginger, crispy wontons, wasabi vinaigrette, and dressing*
- Asian Chopped Chicken Salad
  *without: crispy wontons, vinaigrette, and dressing*
- Miso Side Salad
  *without: miso ginger and side dressing*

# Perkins Restaurant & Bakery

Drink: Water

Farm Fresh Omelets

- Hearty Harvest
  *without: turkey sausage and feta cheese*
- Build-Your-Own
  *without cheese*
  *with two of the following: ham, crimini mushrooms, tomatoes, spinach, fresh broccoli, fresh avocado, onions, green peppers. dry whole wheat toast or fruit on the side*

Perfect Platters

- Potato Pancakes
  *without: butter, applesauce, bacon strips*
  *ask for fresh fruit as a side*

Build-A-Breakfast

- Eggs
  *with grilled ham, fresh fruit, and whole wheat toast (without butter)*

Salads & Soups

*instead of dressing, ask for: lemon, pepper, vinegar, guacamole/avocados, or fresh salsa*

- Southwest Avocado
  *without: cheese, tortilla straws, and dressing*
- The Chopped Cobb
  *without: bacon, feta cheese, and dressing*
- Tomato Basil Soup
  *without croutons*
- Chicken Tortilla Soup
  *without: tortilla strips, cheese, and sour cream*

# Perkins Restaurant & Bakery (2)

Drink: Water

Sides

- Garden Salad
  *without: cheese, croutons, and dressing*
- Fresh Fruit
- Grilled Summer Vegetables
- Fresh Broccoli
- Baked Potato (Plain)
  *without: butter, cheese, bacon, sour cream, etc.*

Comfort Classics

- Grilled Chicken With Mushrooms and Asparagus
  *without: white rice (brown rice okay), vinaigrette, sauce, and sautéed mushrooms (grilled mushrooms instead)*
- Butterball Turkey (see above for sides)
  *without: gravy, cranberry sauce, and dressing*

Burgers

- Hamburger
  *with only: beef patty, lettuce, tomato, egg (ask to be cooked with little to no oil)*
  *without white bread bun (whole wheat/grain bread or lettuce bun instead)*

Half Sandwiches

- Turkey & Avocado
  *without: bacon and aïoli*
- Roast Beef
  *without: French roll (whole wheat bread instead), cheese, and aïoli*

# P.F. Chang's

Drink: Water

## Salads & Soups

*instead of dressing, ask for: lemon, pepper, vinegar, guacamole/avocados, or fresh salsa*

- Asian Caesar Salad (Chicken, Shrimp, or Salmon)
  *without: Parmesan, wonton croutons, and dressing*
- Mandarin Crunch Salad (Chicken, Shrimp, or Salmon)
  *without: crispy rice sticks and vinaigrette/dressing*
- Egg Drop Soup

## Sushi

- Ahi Poke Bowl
  *without: mandarin vinaigrette and wonton crisps*
- Lobster Avocado Roll (if brown rice is available)
  *without: white rice (brown rice instead) and curry aïoli*

## Main Entrees – Chicken, Beef, or Fish

- Chicken, Beef, or Fish With Steamed Broccoli
  *ask for the chicken, beef, or fish to be grilled or cooked with little to no oil. without sauce*
  *with side: steamed brown rice*

## Main Entrees – Vegetarian

- Buddha's Feast
  *without sauce. and ask for vegetables to be steamed or cooked with little to no oil*
  *side: steamed brown rice*

# Poke (General)

- Drink: Water

Base

- Brown Rice
- Spring Mix
- Kale

Fish

- Tuna
- Salmon
- Albacore
- Yellowtail
- Shrimp
- Octopus

Sides

- Crabmeat
- Avocado
- Edamame

Toppings

- Green Onion
- Cucumber
- Sprouts
- Cilantro
- Smelt Eggs
- Red Onion
- Tomato
- Serrano Pepper
- Pineapple

# Pollo Tropical

Drink: Water

## Sides

- Brown Rice
- Black Beans
- Caesar Salad (with Grilled Chicken Breast)
  *without: Caesar dressing, croutons, Parmesan cheese, and Pollo Bites*
- Red Beans
- Brown Rice & Black Beans

## Salads & Soup

*instead of dressing, ask for: lemon, pepper, vinegar, guacamole/avocados, or fresh salsa*

- Mango Chicken Salad (grilled chicken breast)
  *without: candied walnuts, Pollo Bites, and vinaigrette/dressing*
- Caesar Salad (grilled chicken breast)
  *without: caesar dressing, croutons, Parmesan cheese, and Pollo Bites*
- Caribbean Chicken Soup

## TropiChop Bowls

- Chicken or Vegetarian (no sauce)
  *with only: steamed or grilled vegetables (no butter), brown rice, romaine lettuce (no dressing), or ½ lettuce and ½ brown rice + beans, tomatoes, steamed or grilled corn (no butter), and/or peppers*

## Platters

*see above for sides*

- ¼ Fire Grilled Chicken
- ½ Fire Grilled Chicken
- Boneless Chicken Breasts

# Pollo Tropical (2)

Drink: Water

<u>Family Meal</u>

*see above for sides*

- Whole Fire-Grilled Chicken
  *without rolls*

# Popeyes Louisiana Kitchen

Drink: Water

<u>Sides</u>

- Corn On The Cob
  *without butter*
- Red Beans
  *without rice*

Remember:

Many current diets make people think that eating healthily involves counting calories, limiting food consumption, complicated meal preparation, avoiding good protein sources, and/or eliminating carbs. Unfortunately, these common misconceptions about healthy eating lead some to adopt unrealistic and possibly harmful diets. These painful diets rely on dramatic changes of habits and often cause constant feelings of hunger and negative changes in mood.

# Portillo's

Drink: Water

## Sides

- Baked Potato (Plain)
  *without: butter, cheese, bacon, sour cream, etc.*
- Meatball
  *without cheese*
- Garden Side Salad
  *without: cheese, croutons, and vinaigrette/dressing*
- Fruit Cup

## Salads

*instead of dressing, ask for: lemon, pepper, vinegar, guacamole/avocados, or fresh salsa*

- Chopped Salad
  *without: pasta, bacon, cheese, and vinaigrette/dressing*
- Caesar Salad (with Grilled Chicken Breast)
  *without: Caesar dressing, croutons, and Parmesan cheese*
- Greek Salad With Chicken
  *without: cheese and vinaigrette/dressing*
- Garden Side Salad
  *without: cheese, croutons, and vinaigrette/dressing*
- Tuscan Chicken Salad
  *without: dressing, bacon, and walnuts (if candied, otherwise okay)*

## Chicken

- Char-Broiled Chicken Sandwich
  *without: white bread (lettuce bun or whole wheat bun instead) and mayo*

# Portillo's (2)

Drink: Water

<u>Barnelli's Exclusives</u>

- Grilled Filet of Chicken
  *without white bread (wheat and oat bran bun instead) and mayo*
- Grilled Tuna Sandwich
  *without white bread (wheat and oat bran bun instead) and tartar sauce*

Remember:

**Think results and after-effects... to say no to junk food now.**

Thinking about how badly junk food makes the body feel can help stop you from eating junk food in the first place.

# Potbelly Sandwich Shop

Drink: Water

## Sandwiches

*with multigrain or whole wheat bread*
*without white bread*

- Turkey Breast
  *without: cheese and mayo*
- Mediterranean
  *without: hummus and cheese*
- Mediterranean Chicken
  *without: hummus and cheese*
- Smoked Ham
  *without: cheese and mayo*
- Roast Beef
  *without: provolone cheese and mayo*
- Clubby
  *without: bacon, cheese, and ranch*
- Vegetarian
  *without: cheese and mayo*

## Salads

*instead of dressing, ask for: lemon, pepper, vinegar, guacamole/avocados, or fresh salsa*

- Powerhouse
  *without: hummus and dressing*
- Mediterranean
  *without: cheese and dressing*
- Uptown
  *without: cheese, dried cranberries, candied walnuts, and dressing*
- Farmhouse
  *without: bacon, cheese, and dressing*
- A Wreck Salad
  *without: salami, cheese, and dressing*

# Potbelly Sandwich Shop (2)

Drink: Water

Soups

- Classic Tomato
- Garden Vegetable
- Homestyle Chicken Noodle
  *without noodles*

Sides

- Garden Side Salad
  *without dressing*

Remember:
*The Ocinator Restaurant Diet* lists healthy food you can eat at restaurants to help you lose weight the simple way, without the pain of starvation or no-carb diets.

# Qdoba

Drink: Water

## Knockout Tacos

- Drunken Yardbird
  *without: white flour tortilla (soft corn tortilla instead) and cheese*
- Mad Rancher
  *without: white flour tortilla (soft corn tortilla instead) bacon, ranch, and cheese*
- Bohemian Veg
  *without: white flour tortilla (soft corn tortilla instead) and cheese*
- The Gladiator
  *without: white flour tortilla (soft corn tortilla instead), bacon, and cheese*

## Burrito or Bowl

- Grilled Chicken or Steak
  *with: wheat tortilla or bowl + brown rice + black beans + pico de gallo, roasted chile corn, salsa verde, and/or salsa roja + guacamole, shredded lettuce, and/or cilantro*
  *without: cheese and other sauce*

## Soup

- Tortilla Soup
  *with only: chicken, guacamole, and cilantro. (without tortilla strips, cheese, and sour cream)*

# Red Lobster

Drink: Water

## Soups & Salads

*instead of dressing, ask for: lemon, pepper, vinegar, guacamole/avocados, or fresh salsa*

- Classic Caesar Salad
  *without: Parmesan, croutons, and dressing*

## Sides

- Asparagus
  *without butter. steamed or grilled*
- Baked Potato (Plain)
  *without: butter, cheese, bacon, and sour cream*
- Classic Caesar Salad
  *without: Parmesan, croutons, and dressing*
- Broccoli
  *without butter. steamed or grilled*
- Garden Salad
  *without: cheese, croutons, and dressing*

## Shrimp

- Wood-Grilled Shrimp
  *without butter*
- Southwest-Style Tacos (Grilled Shrimp, Grilled Chicken, Fresh Tilapia)
  *without: white flour tortillas (soft corn tortillas instead) and ranch*
- Yucatán Tilapia and Shrimp
  *without: butter, caramelized pineapple (grilled or fresh pineapple instead), and white rice (ask for side from above instead)*

## Shrimp

- Snow Crab Legs
  *without butter*

# Red Lobster (2)

Drink: Water

Land & Sea

- Filet Mignon (6 oz.)
  *without: butter and mashed potatoes (ask for side from above instead)*
- 7 oz. Sirloin
  *without: butter and mashed potatoes (ask for side from above instead)*
- 12 oz. NY Strip
  *without: butter and mashed potatoes (ask for side from above instead)*
- Wood-Grilled Shrimp and Sirloin
  *without: butter, caramelized pineapple (grilled or fresh pineapple instead), and white rice (ask for side from above instead)*

Lobster & Signature Combos

- Wood-Grilled Lobster, Shrimp and Salmon
  *without: butter and white rice (ask for side from above instead)*
- Live Main Lobster
  *see above for sides*
- Rock Lobster Tails
  *without: butter and white rice (ask for side from above instead)*

Fish

- Canadian Walleye (Broiled)
  *without: butter and white rice (ask for side from above instead)*
- Wild-Caught Flounder (Broiled)
  *without: butter and white rice (ask for side from above instead)*

# Red Robin Gourmet Burgers and Brews

Drink: Water

Salads

*instead of dressing, ask for: lemon, pepper, vinegar, guacamole/avocados, or fresh salsa*

- Avo-Cobb-O
  *without: bacon, cheese, garlic toast, and dressing*
- Simply Grilled Chicken Salad
  *without: cheese, garlic toast, and dressing*
- House Salad
  *without: croutons, cheese, and dressing*
- Southwest Salad
  *without: fried jalapeño, cheese, and dressing*
- Mighty Caesar Salad
  *without: Parmesan, dressing, croutons, and garlic toast*
- Side Caesar Salad
  *without: Parmesan, dressing, croutons, and garlic toast*

Sides

- Side Salad
  *without: croutons, cheese, and dressing*
- Steamed Broccoli
- Black Beans

Other Fun On A Bun

- Simply Grilled Chicken
  *without: cheese, sauce, and white bread (ask for a whole wheat or lettuce bun instead)*

# Red Robin Gourmet Burgers and Brews (2)

Drink: Water

Gourmet Burgers

- Veggie Burger
  *without: white bread bun (whole wheat/grain or lettuce bun instead), cheese, Parmesan-sprinkled mushrooms, and sauce*

Entrées

- Ensenada Chicken
  *without: cheese, tortilla strips, and ranch*
- Sear-ious Salmon
  *without coleslaw. ask for salmon to be cooked without butter and little to no oil*

Remember:
With over 1,000 healthy menu options, this book helps busy folks like you to eat on the go, healthily, and without the pain that many other diets produce. It is an ongoing solution to promote long-term health.

# Ruby Tuesday

Drink: Water

## Salads

*instead of dressing, ask for: lemon, pepper, vinegar, guacamole/avocados, or fresh salsa*

- Endless Garden Bar
  *without: dressing, cheese, dried cranberries, crispy onions, candied walnuts, crispy Parmesan chips, hummus, pasta salad, potato salad, ham & pea pasta, croutons, bacon, crackers, and olive oil*

## Soups

- Roasted Tomato
- Garden Vegetable

## Burgers & Sandwiches

*without white bread (whole wheat/grain or lettuce bun/bread instead)*

- Triple Prime Burger
  *without: sauce, mayo, cheese, and fries (garden bar instead)*
- Avocado Turkey Burger
  *without: bacon, sauce, mayo, cheese, and fries (garden bar instead)*
- Grilled Chicken Sandwich
  *without: sauce, mayo, cheese, and fries (garden bar instead)*
- Avocado Grilled Chicken
  *without: sauce, mayo, cheese, pickle chips, and fries (garden bar instead)*

## Chicken & Pasta

*see below for sides*

- Chicken Fresco
  *without: lemon butter and balsamic vinaigrette*
- Chicken 'Bella
  *without: Parmesan cream sauce and lemon butter*
  *see below for sides*

# Ruby Tuesday (2)

Drink: Water

<u>Seafood & Steaks</u>

- Blackened Tilapia
  *without butter. see below for sides*
- Grilled Salmon
  *without: sauce or butter. see below for sides*
- Rib Eye
  *without butter. see below for sides*
- 6 oz. or 8 oz. Top Sirloin
  *without butter. ask chef to cook with very little oil. see below for sides*

<u>Sides</u>

- Garden Salad
  *without: cheese, croutons, and dressing*
- Steamed Broccoli
- Baked Potato (Plain)
  *without: cheese, sour cream, and butter*
- Grilled Zucchini
  *without butter*
- Sweet Potato (Plain)
  *without: butter, sugar, marshmallows, candied walnuts, and jam*

# Ruth's Chris Steak House

Drink: Water

## Steaks & Chops

*ask for meat to be cooked without butter and with little to no oil*

- Filet
- Cowboy Ribeye
- New York Strip
- Petite Filet & Shrimp
- Ribeye
- T-Bone
- Porterhouse For Two
- Petite Filet
- Petite Ribeye
- Lamb Chops
- Tomahawk Ribeye
- Bone-In Filet
- Bone-In New York Strip

## Entrée Complements

- Shrimp
  *without butter*
- Lobster Tail
  *without butter*

## Seafood & Specialties

- Chilean Sea Bass
  *without butter. ask for sweet potato and pineapple hash to be cooked with little to no oil*
- Vegetarian Plate
  *without: cheese and butter. ask to be cooked with little to no oil*

# Ruth's Chris Steak House (2)

Drink: Water

Appetizers & Sides

- Roasted Brussel Sprouts
  *without: butter and bacon. ask to be cooked with little to no oil*
- Grilled Asparagus
  *without: butter and sauce. ask to be cooked with little to no oil*
- Fresh Broccoli
- Baked Potato (Plain)
  *without: cheese, sour cream, bacon, and butter*

Soups & Salads

*instead of dressing, ask for: lemon, pepper, vinegar, guacamole/avocados, or fresh salsa*

*ask for meat to be cooked without butter and with little to no oil*

- Steak House Salad
  *without: croutons and dressing*
- Ruth's Chop Salad
  *without: bacon, cheese, dressing, and crispy onions*
- Lettuce Wedge
  *without: bacon, cheese, and dressing*
- Harvest Salad
  *without: bacon, dried cranberries, cheese, Cajun pecans, vinaigrette, and dressing*
- Fresh Broccoli
- Baked Potato (Plain)
  *without fixings (cheese, butter, sour cream, bacon, etc.)*

# Schlotzsky's

Drink: Water

## Sandwiches

- Fresh Veggie
  *without: cheese and dressing. with whole wheat/grain bread*
- Smoked Turkey Breast
  *without: sourdough (whole wheat/grain bread instead) and mayonnaise*
- Fiesta Chicken Sandwich
  *without: sourdough (whole wheat/grain bread instead), cheese, and chipotle mayo*
- Turkey & Guacamole
  *without: sauce or cheese. with whole wheat/grain bread*
- Fiesta Chicken
  *without: jalapeño cheese bun (whole wheat/grain bread instead), cheese, and chipotle mayo*
- Angus Roast Beef
  *without: sourdough bun (whole wheat/grain bread instead), cheese, pickles, mayo, and sauce*

## Soups

- Tomato Basil
  *without cheese*
- Garden Vegetable
  *without: cheese, dried cranberries, candied pecans, croutons, garlic breadstick, and dressing*
- Chicken Tortilla
  *without: cheese and tortilla strips*

# Schlotzsky's (2)

Drink: Water

<u>Salads</u>

*instead of dressing, ask for: lemon, pepper, vinegar, guacamole/avocados, or fresh salsa*

- Fresh Kale & Grilled Chicken Salad
  *without: cheese, dried cranberries, candied pecans, garlic breadstick, and dressing*
- Cranberry, Apple, Pecan & Chicken Salad
  *without: cheese, dried cranberries, candied pecans, croutons, garlic breadstick, and dressing*
- Southwestern Chicken Salad
  *without: cheese, tortilla strips, breadstick, and dressing*
- Turkey Avocado Cobb Salad
  *without: cheese, bacon, croutons, breadstick, and dressing*
- Chicken Caesar Salad
  *without: cheese, croutons, breadstick, and dressing*

Remember:

While trendy diets and workout programs grow in popularity, the obesity rate is not decreasing. In fact, obesity related conditions like heart disease, stroke, type 2 diabetes and certain types of cancer continue to be some of the leading causes of preventable, premature death.

Helping restaurant-goers eat a sound meal is a need that was largely unmet by diet books… until now.

# Sharky's

Drink: Water

Get It Naked

- Organic Roasted Vegetable Bowl
  *without pesto (lemon, pico, or guacamole instead)*
  Naked Chicken Fajita Bowl
  *ask for fajitas to be cooked with little to no oil*
- Naked Sharky's Chicken Salad
  *without: dressing (lemon, pico, or guacamole instead)*
- Wild Salmon "Lite" Burrito
  *without aïoli*
- Santa Fe "Lite" Burrito
  *without cheese*

Power Plates

*with any of the following: organic poblano brown rice, organic quinoa with veggies, grilled veggies, organic black beans, organic pinto beans, steamed broccoli, organic Yucatan yams, organic roasted vegetables*

- All Natural Chicken Breast
- All Natural Angus Steak
- Wild Caught Salmon
- Wild Caught Fish
- Shrimp

Tacos

*with soft corn tortillas (without flour tortillas)*

- Original
- California
  *without cheese*
- Organic Tofu & Veggies
- Wild Caught Fish or Shrimp
  *without: cheese and sauce*

# Sharky's (2)

Drink: Water

## Burritos

*with low-fat whole wheat tortilla (without white flour tortilla)*

- Fiesta (Chicken or Steak)
  *without: white rice (brown rice instead), cheese, and sour cream (non-fat sour cream is okay)*
- Sharky's (Chicken or Steak)
  *without white rice (brown rice instead)*
- Santa Fe (Chicken or Steak)
  *without cheese*
- Wild Caught Fish or Shrimp
  *without: white rice (brown rice instead), cheese, and sauce*
- Organic Tofu & Veggies

## Salads

*instead of dressing, ask for: lemon, pepper, vinegar, guacamole/avocados, or fresh salsa*

*optional add-ons: chicken, steak, wild caught salmon, grilled shrimp*

- Summer Harvest
  *without: dressing, raisins, and cheese*
- Sharky's Chicken
  *without: tortilla strips, rice noodles, and dressing*
- Numex Caesar
  *without: croutons, tortilla strips, cheese, and dressing*
- Sharky's Quinoa
  *without vinaigrette*
- Side Salad
  *without: croutons and cheese*

## Soup

- Chicken Tortilla
  *without: tortilla strips, cheese, and sour cream (non-fat sour cream is okay)*

# Smashburger

Drink: Water

<u>Beef, Chicken, Turkey, or Black Bean Patty</u>

*on a multigrain bun*

*ask for meat and bread not to be buttered*

- Classic
  *without: white bread bun, cheese, mayo, and sauce*
- Avocado Club
  *without: white bread bun, cheese, mayo, and sauce*
- Spinach, Cucumber & Goat Cheese
  *without: white bread bun, cheese, mayo, and sauce*
- Create Your Own
  *with: multigrain bun, avocado, grilled mushrooms, guacamole, cucumbers, spinach, lettuce, tomatoes, and onion*
  *without: white bread bun, sauce and dressing, cheese, and fries*

<u>Salads</u>

*instead of dressing, ask for: lemon, pepper, vinegar, guacamole/avocados, or fresh salsa*

- Classic Cobb Salad
  *without: bacon, cheese, ranch, and dressing*
- Spinach, Cucumber & Goat Cheese Salad
  *without: cheese, vinaigrette, and dressing*

# Sonic

Drink: Water

Chicken

- Classic Grilled Chicken
  *without: white bread (lettuce bun instead), cheese, mayo, sauce, and fries*

# Steak 'n Shake

Drink: Water

Specialty Steakburgers

- Fresh Guacamole
  *without: white bread (lettuce bun instead), cheese, mayo, sauce, and fries*

Specialty Sandwiches

- Grilled Chicken Sandwich
  *without: white bread (lettuce bun instead), cheese, mayo, sauce, and fries*

Salads

- Fresh Guacamole
  *without: cheese, croutons, and dressing*
- Grilled Chicken Salad
  *without: cheese, croutons, and dressing*

# Subway

Drink: Water

<u>Sandwiches & Flatbreads</u>

*with 9-Grain Wheat, Multigrain Flatbread, or Rye*

*+ veggies*

*+ (optional) guacamole*

*+ (optional) red wine vinegar*

*without cheese, bacon, pepperoni, sauce, and dressing*

- Oven Roasted Chicken
- Black Forest Ham
- Roast Beef
- Rotisserie-Style Chicken
- Turkey Breast
- Veggie Delite

<u>Salads</u>

*+ veggies*

*+ (optional) guacamole*

*+ (optional) red wine vinegar*

*without cheese, bacon, pepperoni, sauce, and dressing*

- Oven Roasted Chicken
- Black Forest Ham
- Roast Beef
- Rotisserie-Style Chicken
- Turkey Breast
- Veggie Delite

# Taco Bell

Drink: Water

<u>Power Menu</u>

*instead of dressing, ask for: lemon, pepper, vinegar, guacamole/avocados, or fresh salsa*

- Power Bowl (Chicken)
  *without: cheese, rice, ranch, sauce, dressing, and sour cream*
  *(optional add-ons) only: lettuce, onions, tomatoes, and beans*
- Power Bowl
  *without: cheese, rice, ranch, sauce, dressing, and sour cream*
  *(optional add-ons) only: lettuce, onions, tomatoes, and beans*

<u>Sides</u>

- Black Beans
  *(optional add-ons and upgrades) only: chicken, lettuce, onions, tomatoes, beans, guacamole, and onions*

Remember:
*The Ocinator Restaurant Diet* is intended to help users lose body fat. To help you sculpt abs and other muscles, we recommend the Ocinator Fitness Program as the ideal companion to this book. Ocinator workouts are simple and do not aim for sweat and exhaustion. On the contrary, Ocinator workouts were designed to minimize workout time (20 minutes/day) and pain so that users can realistically maintain results and a positive long-term change in fitness lifestyle.

# Taco Cabana

Drink: Water

## Breakfast

- Egg Taco
  *without: flour tortilla (soft corn tortilla instead), cheese, bacon, and chorizo*

## Tacos

- Flame-Grilled USDA Choice Steak Street Tacos
  *with soft corn tortilla*
- Shredded Chicken Taco
  *without: flour tortilla (soft corn tortilla instead) and cheese*
- Black Bean Taco
  *without: flour tortilla (soft corn tortilla instead) and rice*

## Bowls

- Bowl with No Shell (Grilled Chicken or Steak)
  *without: rice, sour cream, and cheese*

## Sides

- Refried Beans
  *without cheese*
- Black Beans
  *without cheese*
- Guacamole

# Taco John's

Drink: Water

Tacos

- Street Tacos (Sirloin steak or Grilled Chicken
  *without: flour tortillas (soft corn tortillas instead), garlic lime sauce, and cheese. if soft corn tortillas are not available, ask for more lettuce as a substitute*

Sides

*instead of dressing, ask for: lemon, pepper, vinegar, guacamole/avocados, or fresh salsa*

- Refried Beans
  *without cheese*
- Side Salad
  *without: cheese and dressing*

Remember:
Both *The Ocinator Restaurant Diet* and Ocinator Fitness aim to make obtaining and maintaining long-term fitness results simple and realistic.
See Ocinator.com for more details.
Now… it's time to enjoy all your new restaurant menu options and feel great!

# Texas de Brazil Churrascaria

Drink: Water

## Meats

*don't eat the meat fat*

- Pinanha
- Leg of Lamb
- Lamb Chops
- Garlic Picanha
- Filet Mignon
- Flank Steak

## Salad Area

*without dressing and vinaigrette. instead, ask for: lemon, pepper, vinegar, guacamole/avocados, or fresh salsa*

- Tomato Slices
- Steamed Asparagus
- Malgueta Peppers
- Heart of Palm
- Romaine Lettuce
- Ceviche Onions
- Roasted Red & Yellow Peppers
- Tabbouleh
- Couscous Salad
- Marinated Artichoke Hearts
- Roasted Jalapeños
- Sushi (brown rice) *without white rice*
- Smoked Salmon
- Peppadew Peppers
- Pepperoncini
- Sun-Dried Cherry Tomatoes
- Kalamata Olives
- Cherry Tomatoes

## Hot Items

- Moqueca Fish Stew
- Brazilian Black Beans (if cooked without bacon)

# Texas Roadhouse

Drink: Water

## Salads

*instead of dressing, ask for: lemon, pepper, vinegar, guacamole/avocados, or fresh salsa*

- Grilled Chicken Salad
  *without: cheese, bacon, croutons, and dressing*
- Steakhouse Filet Salad
  *without: cheese, bacon, croutons, and dressing. ask for steak to be cooked without butter and with little to no oil*
- House Salad
  *without: cheese, croutons, and dressing*
- Caesar Salad
  *without: cheese, croutons, and dressing*
- Chicken Caesar Salad
  *without: cheese, croutons, and dressing*

## Sides

- Fresh Vegetables
  *without butter*
- House Salad
  *without: cheese, croutons, and dressing*
- Caesar Salad
  *without: cheese, croutons, and dressing*
- Baked Potato (Plain)
  *without: cheese, bacon, butter, sour cream, etc.*
- Sweet Potato (Plain)
  *without: marshmallows and caramel sauce*
- Green Beans (Steamed)
  *without: butter and oil*

## Country Dinners

- Country Vegetable Plate
  *see above for sides*

# Texas Roadhouse (2)

Drink: Water

## Chicken Specialties

*see above for sides*

- Oven Roasted Half Chicken
  *without: cheese, bacon, croutons, and dressing*

## Steaks

*ask for steak to be cooked without butter and with little to no oil*

*see above for sides*

- Ft. Worth Ribeye
- Dallas Filet
- USDA Choice Sirloin
- New York Strip
- Porterhouse T-Bone
- Steak Kabob
  *without white rice*

## Dockside Favorites

*see above for sides*

- Grilled Shrimp
  *without: butter and white rice (ask for fresh vegetables instead). ask for shrimp to be cooked with little to no oil*
- Grilled Salmon
  *without butter. ask for salmon to be cooked with little to no oil*

## Burgers & Sandwiches

*see above for sides*

- Chicken Sandwich
  *without: white bread bun (whole wheat/grain or lettuce bun instead) sautéed mushrooms (grilled instead), and cheese*
- Burger
  *without: white bread bun (whole wheat/grain or lettuce bun instead), bacon, sautéed mushrooms (grilled instead), and cheese*

# TGI Fridays

Drink: Water

## Sides

- House Salad
  *without: cheese, croutons, and dressing*
- Caesar Salad
  *without: cheese, croutons, Parmesan crisps, and dressing*
- Super Veggies

## Salads & Soups

*instead of dressing, ask for: lemon, pepper, vinegar, guacamole/avocados, and/or fresh salsa*

- House Salad
  *without: cheese, croutons, dressing, and breadstick*
- Caesar Salad
  *without: cheese, croutons, Parmesan crisps, dressing, and breadstick*
- Strawberry Fields Salad With Grilled Chicken
  *without: cheese, Parmesan, glazed pecans, dressing/vinaigrette, and breadstick*
- Caesar Salad With Grilled Chicken
  *without: cheese, croutons, Parmesan crisps, dressing, and breadstick*
- Million Dollar Cobb
  *without: bacon, cheese, Parmesan, dressing, vinaigrette/dressing, and breadstick*

## Appetizers

- Grilled Wings
  *without: sauce and dressing*

# TGI Fridays (2)

Drink: Water

## Burgers

*see above for sides*

- Turkey Burger
  *without: white bread (lettuce or whole wheat bun instead), sauce, and fries*
- Burger
  *without: white bread bun (whole wheat/grain or lettuce bun instead), bacon, sautéed mushrooms (grilled instead), and cheese*

## Sandwiches

*see above for sides*

- Turkey + Avocado
  *without: white bread (lettuce or whole wheat bun instead), bacon, Swiss, sauce, pesto, and fries*

## Chicken, Seafood & Pasta

*see above for sides*

- Dragon-Glaze Salmon
  *without: glaze and white rice (brown rice or more veggies instead)*
- Dragon-Glaze Chicken
  *without: glaze and white rice (brown rice or more veggies instead)*

## Steaks & Ribs

*don't eat the meat fat*

- Center-Cut Sirloin
  *without: butter and mashed potatoes (brown rice or more veggies instead)*
- New York Strip
  *without: butter and mashed potatoes (brown rice or more veggies instead)*

# The Capital Grille

Drink: Water

## Salads

*instead of dressing, ask for: lemon, pepper, vinegar, guacamole/avocados, and/or fresh salsa*

- Maine Lobster Salad
  *without: vinaigrette/dressing*
- Caesar Salad With All-Natural Chicken Breast
  *without: cheese, croutons, Parmesan crisps, and dressing*
- Seared Salmon With Avocado, Mango, and Tomato Salad
  *without: champagne vinaigrette/dressing*
- The Capital Grille "Cobb" Salad With Sliced Tenderloin
  *without vinaigrette/dressing*
- Seared Tuna Salad
  *ask for tuna to be cooked with little no oil*
  *without vinaigrette/dressing*

## Burgers and Sandwiches

*without Parmesan truffle fries or chips. see above for sides to ask for instead*

- Lobster and Crab Burger
  *without: white bread bun (ask for whole wheat/grain bun or lettuce bun instead) and tartar sauce*
- Ribeye Steak Sandwich
  *without: white bread bun (ask for whole wheat/grain bun or lettuce bun instead), sauce, caramelized onions (grilled onions instead), and Havarti*
- Maine Lobster Roll
  *without: brioche bun (ask for whole wheat/grain bun or lettuce bun instead), tartar sauce, bacon, and cheese*

# The Capital Grille (2)

Drink: Water

## Plates

*with field greens salad, no croutons, cheese, dressing and vinaigrette instead of dressing, ask for: lemon, pepper, vinegar, guacamole/avocados, and/or fresh salsa*

- Seared Salmon with Asparagus and Shiitakes
  *ask for salmon, asparagus, and shiitakes to be cooked with little to no oil*
  *without parsnip purée*
- Mini Tenderloin Sandwiches
  *without: white bread bun (ask for whole wheat/grain bun or lettuce bun instead), sauce, caramelized onions (grilled onions instead), cheese, and Parmesan truffle fries*
- Grilled Breast of Chicken
  *without: caramelized onions (grilled onions instead)*
  *ask for baby potatoes to be cooked without oil*

## Entrées

*with steamed or grilled green beans (not French) or a salad without cheese, croutons, and dressing/vinaigrette*

- Filet Mignon 8 oz
- Bone-In Dry Aged NY Strip
  *without: cheese, croutons, Parmesan crisps, and dressing*
- Sushi-Grade Sesame Seared Tuna
  *ask for tuna to be cooked with little to no oil*
  *without: white rice (ask more green beans or salad instead) and sauces*
- Roasted Swordfish
  *without gratin (ask more green beans or salad instead)*
- Sliced Filet Mignon
  *without cipollini mushrooms. ask for vegetables to be cooked with little to no oil*

# The Cheesecake Factory

Drink: Water

## Appetizer Salads

- Tossed Green Salad
  *without: croutons and vinaigrette/dressing*
- French Country Salad
  *without: goat cheese, candied pecans, and vinaigrette/dressing*
- Fresh Vegetable Salad
  *without: cheese and vinaigrette/dressing*
- Factory Chopped Salad
  *without: bacon, cheese, and vinaigrette/dressing*

## Salads

*instead of dressing, ask for: lemon, pepper, vinegar, guacamole/avocados, and/or fresh salsa*

- Caesar Salad
  *without: croutons, cheese, and dressing*
- Sheila's Chicken and Avocado Salad
  *without: tortilla strips and vinaigrette/dressing*
- Chinese Chicken Salad
  *without: white rice noodles, crisp wontons, and vinaigrette/dressing*
- Chicken, Mango, and Avocado Salad
  *without: crispy wontons and vinaigrette/dressing*
- Chipotle Grilled Shrimp Salad
  *without: cheese and vinaigrette/dressing*
- Santa Fe Salad
  *without: cheese, tortilla strips, and vinaigrette/dressing*
- Cobb Salad
  *without: bacon, cheese, and vinaigrette/dressing*
- Seared Tuna Tataki Salad
  *without vinaigrette/dressing*

# The Cheesecake Factory (2)

Drink: Water

<u>Appetizers</u>

- Fire-Roasted Fresh Artichoke
  *without garlic dip*
- Guacamole
  *without tortilla chips (ask for soft corn tortillas instead if available)*

<u>Small Plates & Snacks</u>

- Little House Salad
  *without vinaigrette/dressing*
- Greek Salad
  *without: cheese and vinaigrette/dressing*
- Edamame
  *without gratin (ask more green beans or salad instead)*

<u>"Super" Foods</u>

- Avocado Toast (if whole grain/wheat bread is available)
  *without: white bread (ask for whole wheat/grain bread instead) and olive oil*
- California Guacamole Salad
  *without: crispy tortillas, feta cheese, and dressing/vinaigrette (guacamole is okay)*
- Wellness Salad
  *without: roasted pear, sunflower seeds, and vinaigrette/dressing*
- Kale and Quinoa Salad
  *without: Parmesan cheese, sunflower seeds, and vinaigrette/dressing*
- Vegan Cobb Salad
  *without: sunflower seeds and vinaigrette/dressing*
- Almond-Crusted Salmon Salad
  *ask for salmon to be cooked with little to no oil*
  *without: dried cranberries and vinaigrette/dressing*

# The Cheesecake Factory (3)

Drink: Water

## Glamburgers & Sandwiches

*without fries. instead, ask for green salad without dressing, croutons, and cheese*

- Grilled Turkey Burger
  *without sauce/dressing*
- Veggie Burger
  *without: cheese, garlic aïoli, and sauce/dressing*
- Grilled Chicken And Avocado Club
  *without: white bread (whole wheat/grain or lettuce bun instead), Swiss, mayo, and fries*
- Southwest Chicken Sandwich
  *without: white bread (whole wheat/grain or lettuce bun instead) and chipotle mayo*
- Impossible Burger
  *without: white bread (whole wheat/grain or lettuce bun instead) and sauce*

## Specialties

- Chicken Enchiladas
  *without: cheese (on enchiladas and beans) and cilantro rice (more corn without butter instead)*
- Baja Chicken Tacos
  *without: cheese (in tacos and on beans) and cilantro rice (more corn without butter instead)*
- Baja Chicken Tacos
  *without: cheese (in tacos and on beans) and cilantro rice (more corn without butter instead)*

# The Cheesecake Factory (4)

Drink: Water

Steaks, Chops, Fish & Seafood

*without butter and little to no oil*

- Carne Asada
  *without: sauce, white rice (ask for more corn without butter and cheese instead), sautéed vegetables (ask for grilled vegetables with little to no oil instead), and butter and cheese (on corn)*
- Chargrilled Bone-In New York Steak
  *without mashed potatoes (more vegetables instead)*
- Grilled Rib-Eye Steak
  *without mashed potatoes (more vegetables instead)*
- Filet Mignon
  *without mashed potatoes (more vegetables instead)*
- Fresh Grilled Salmon
  *without: sauce and mashed potatoes (more broccoli/vegetables instead)*
- Herb Crusted Filet of Salmon
  *without: lemon sauces and mashed potatoes (more asparagus/vegetables instead)*

Skinnylicious Small Plates and Appetizers

- Greek Salad
  *without: feta cheese and vinaigrette/dressing*
- Little House Salad
  *without vinaigrette/dressing*
- Skinnylicious Grilled Artichoke
  *without lemon-garlic aïoli*
- Chicken Lettuce Wrap Tacos (Asian or Mexican)
  *without: white rice noodles and sauce/dressing on chicken*
- Ahi Tartare
  *without soy-ginger sesame sauce*

# The Cheesecake Factory (5)

Drink: Water

Skinnylicious Salads

*instead of dressing, ask for: lemon, pepper, vinegar, guacamole/avocados, and/or fresh salsa*

- Skinnylicious Tossed Green Salad
  *without: croutons and dressing*
- Skinnylicious French Country Salad
  *without: goat cheese, candied pecans, and vinaigrette/dressing*
- Skinnylicious Caesar Salad
  *without: croutons, cheese, and dressing*
- Skinnylicious Fresh Vegetable Salad
  *without: cheese and vinaigrette/dressing*
- Skinnylicious Factory Chopped Salad
  *without: bacon, cheese, and vinaigrette/dressing*
- Skinnylicious Asian Chicken Salad
  *without: white rice noodles, crisp wontons, and vinaigrette/dressing*
- Skinnylicious Mexican Tortilla Salad
  *without: crispy corn tortilla (soft corn tortillas instead), cheese, tortilla strips, avocado cream sauce (plain avocados instead), sour cream, and vinaigrette/dressing*
- Skinnylicious Seared Tuna Tataki Salad
  *ask for tuna to be seared with little to no oil*
  *without wasabi vinaigrette*

# The Cheesecake Factory (6)

Drink: Water

Skinnylicious Specialties

*without fries. ask for green salad without dressing, croutons, and cheese instead*

- Skinnylicious Hamburger
  *without: white bread bun (whole wheat/grain or lettuce bun instead), pickles, and mayonnaise*
- Skinnylicious Veggie Burger
  *without: white bread bun (whole wheat/grain or lettuce bun instead), pickles, and mayonnaise*
- Skinnylicious Grilled Turkey Burger
  *without: white bread bun (whole wheat/grain or lettuce bun instead) and mayonnaise*
- Skinnylicious Turkey & Avocado Sandwich
  *without: white bread bun (whole wheat/grain or lettuce bun instead), bacon, and mayonnaise*
- Skinnylicious Soft Tacos
  *without: crema and escabeche vegetables (grilled or steamed vegetables instead)*
- Skinnylicious Chicken Enchiladas
  *without: cheese and escabeche vegetables (grilled or steamed vegetables instead)*
- Skinnylicious Tuscan Chicken
  *without: balsamic vinaigrette and sauce*
- Skinnylicious Grilled Salmon
  *without: balsamic vinaigrette and sauce*

# The Cheesecake Factory (7)

Drink: Water

Eggs & Omelettes

*ask for eggs to be cooked without butter and with little to no oil*

- Farm Fresh Eggs
  *with: tomatoes or whole wheat/grain toast*
- Factory Huevos Rancheros
  *without: cheese (on eggs and beans), crispy tortillas (soft corn tortillas instead), and sour cream*
- Factory Create An Omelette
  *with four of the following: ham, avocado, peppers, mushrooms, asparagus, spinach, bell peppers, tomato, red or green onions*
- California Omelette
  *without cheese (in tacos and on beans), chorizo, and sour cream*
- Spinach and Mushroom Omelette
  *without: cheese (in tacos and on beans), sautéed mushrooms (grilled instead), bacon, and sour cream*
- Breakfast Tacos
  *without: cheese (in tacos and on beans), and sour cream*

Remember:

**Small changes make a huge difference.**

It might seem like the difference between white bread and whole grain bread, water and lemonade, dressing and no dressing, are of little significance. False. These small changes are what allow you to lose fat without spending all day doing cardio.

# The Habit Burger Grill

Drink: Water

## Charburgers

*without fries*

- Charburger
  *without: white bread bun (whole wheat bun instead), caramelized onions, pickles, and sauce/dressing*
- Double Charburger
  *without: white bread bun (whole wheat bun instead), caramelized onions, pickles, mayo, and sauce/dressing*
- Santa Barbara Char
  *without: white bread bun (whole wheat bun instead), cheese, caramelized onions, pickles, and sauce/dressing*

## Salads

*instead of dressing, ask for: lemon, pepper, vinegar, guacamole/avocados, and/or fresh salsa*

- Garden Salad
  *without: croutons, cheese, and dressing/vinaigrette*
- Grilled Chicken Salad
  *without: croutons, cheese, and dressing/vinaigrette*
- Grilled Chicken Caesar
  *without: Caesar dressing, croutons, cheese, and dressing/vinaigrette*
- Super Food Salad
  *without: Craisins, cheese, and dressing/vinaigrette*
- Santa Barbara Cobb
  *without: bacon, cheese, croutons, and dressing/vinaigrette*
- Caesar Salad
  *without: Caesar dressing, croutons, cheese, and dressing/vinaigrette*

# The Habit Burger Grill (2)

Drink: Water

Sandwiches

*instead of dressing, ask for: lemon, pepper, vinegar, guacamole/avocados, and/or fresh salsa*

- Veggie Burger
  *without sweet mustard*

Sides

- Side Caesar Salad
  *without: Caesar dressing, croutons, cheese, and dressing/vinaigrette*
- Side Salad
  *without: cheese (on eggs and beans), crispy tortillas (soft corn tortillas instead), and sour cream*

# Tim Hortons

Drink: Water

Sandwiches

*without white bread bun (lettuce bun instead), bacon, cheese, and sauce/dressing*

- Turkey
- Ham

Soups

- Hearty Vegetable
- Chicken Noodle
  *without noodles*

Breakfast

- Homestyle Oatmeal (Mixed Berries or Plain)
  *without added sugar*

# Tropical Smoothie Cafe

Drink: Water

## Bowls

- Baja Chicken Bowl
  *without: pickled red onion, cheese, and dressing/vinaigrette*
- Supergreen Caesar Chicken Bowl
  *without: Parmesan, Parmesan crisps, and Caesar dressing*
- Santa Barbara Char
  *without: white bun (whole wheat or lettuce bun instead), cheese, caramelized onions, pickles, and sauce/dressing*

## Superfood Smoothies

*without any added sugar*

- Acai Berry Boost
- Avocolada
- Chia Banana Boost
  *without peanut butter*
- Chia Banana Max
  *without peanut butter*
- Detox Island Green
  *without natural sweetener*
- Health Nut
- Acai Island Green
- Lean Machine
- Muscle Blaster
- Orange Ginger Glow
- Pomegranate Plunge
- Triple Berry Oat
  *without Splenda*

# Tropical Smoothie Café (2)

Drink: Water

Classic Smoothies

*without any added sugar or juice (fruit only)*

- Blueberry Bliss
- Jetty Punch
- Kiwi Quencher
  *without peanut butter*
- Mango Magic
  *without peanut butter*
- Paradise Point
  *without natural sweetener*
- Peaches 'N Silk
- Strawberry Limeade

Sandwiches

*without fries. ask for green salad without dressing, croutons, and cheese instead*

- Turkey
  *with: 9-grain bread, lettuce, and tomatoes*
  *without: bacon, cheese, and honey dijon*

# Village Inn

Drink: Water

Dinner

- Lemon Artichoke Chicken
  *without: white rice, lemon-parsley butter sauce, and sautéed spinach (ask for grilled spinach without oil instead)*
  *ask for an extra side from below instead*
- Top Sirloin
  *without: butter, mashed potatoes, and gravy*
  *(ask for two other sides from below instead)*
- Slow Roasted Turkey
  *without: stuffing, mashed potatoes, and gravy*
  *(ask for two other sides from below instead)*

Lunch

*with fresh fruit, side salad (see Sides details below), or tomato basil soup*

- Turkey Avocado Sandwich
  *without: bacon, cheese, and mayo*
- Burger
  *without: white bread bun (wheat bread bun or lettuce bun instead), cheese, bacon, onion rings, and dressing*
  *with: tomato, lettuce, fresh onions*
- All-White Meat Chicken Breast Burger
  *without: white bread bun (wheat bread bun or lettuce bun instead), cheese, bacon, onion rings, and dressing*
  *with: tomato, lettuce, fresh onions*
- Classy Cobb Salad
  *without: bacon, cheese, and dressing/vinaigrette*
- Celebrity Chef Salad
  *without: cheese, croutons, and dressing/vinaigrette*
- Southwest Salad
  *without: crispy tortilla strips and dressing/vinaigrette*

# Village Inn (2)

Drink: Water or Low-Fat Milk

## Sides

*instead of dressing, ask for: lemon, pepper, vinegar, guacamole/avocados, and/or fresh salsa*

- Tomato Basil Soup
- Side Garden Salad
  *without: cheese, croutons, dressing, and dressing/vinaigrette*
- Fresh Fruit
- Fresh Broccoli
- Green Beans
  *without butter*
- Corn
  *without butter*

## Breakfast

*ask for eggs to be cooked without butter and with little to no oil*

- Top Sirloin & Eggs
  *ask for eggs and sirloin to be cooked without butter*
  *without: pancakes and hash browns*
- California Skillet
  *ask for skillet to be cooked with little to no oil*
  *without: bacon, cheese, and hollandaise. (ask for potatoes to be cooked without oil and ask for eggs to be cooked without butter)*

# Village Inn (3)

Drink: Water or Low-Fat Milk

## Omelettes

*without buttermilk pancakes and hash browns. multigrain pancakes (ask to be cooked with little to no sugar) instead*

- Denver Omelette
  *without cheese*
- Fresh Spinach & Bacon Omelette
  *without: bacon, cheese, and hollandaise sauce*
- Garden Veggie Omelette
  *without cheese*
- Create Your Own Omelette
  *without cheese*
  *with any of the following: onions, mushrooms, fresh spinach, tomatoes, broccoli, green peppers, artichokes, ham, and avocado*
- Tres Huevos Rancheros
  *without: cheese (on eggs and beans), crispy corn tortillas (soft corn tortillas instead), pork green chili, and sour cream*
- Fruit & Nut Multigrain Pancakes
  *ask to be cooked with little to no sugar*
  *without: jam, jelly, preserves, and syrup*

## Breakfast Sides

- Fresh Fruit
- Cinnamon Apples
  *without added sugar*
- Quaker Oatmeal (plain)
  *without added sugar*
- Whole Grain/Wheat Toast (if available)

# Waffle House

Drink: Water or Low-Fat Milk

## Breakfast

- ask for eggs cooked without butter and with little to no oil and only get toast if whole wheat/grain bread is available

## Toddle House Omelettes

- Ham
  *without cheese*
- Fiesta
  *without cheese*

## Steak & Eggs

- T-Bone & Eggs
  *without cheese*
- Steak & Eggs
  *without: bacon, cheese, and hollandaise sauce*
- Grilled Chicken& Eggs
  *without cheese*

## Eggs

*ask for eggs to be cooked without butter and with little to no oil*

- 3 Eggs
- 2 Eggs
- 1 Egg

# Waffle House (2)

Drink: Water or Low-Fat Milk

<u>Lunch & Dinner</u>

*garden salad without croutons, cheese, and dressing, without hash browns and white bread toast (get whole wheat/grain bread without butter if available). ask for more salad instead*

- T-Bone Steak
- Sirloin
- Grilled Chicken
  *without cheese*
- Grilled Chicken Sandwich
  *without: white bread bun (whole wheat/grain bun or lettuce bun instead), cheese, bacon, and sauce/dressing*

We hope this book will help you enjoy eating out at the most popular U.S. chain restaurants. And that the food recommendations within will help you look and feel as fit and fantastic as you deserve to be.

# Wendy's

Drink: Water

## Chicken

- Grilled Chicken Sandwich
  *without: white bread (whole wheat/grain bun or lettuce bun instead), honey mustard, and cheese*

## Fresh-Made Salads

*instead of dressing, ask for: lemon, pepper, vinegar, guacamole/avocados, and/or fresh salsa*

- Harvest Salad
  *without: cheese, dried cranberries, brown sugar walnuts, bacon, and dressing/vinaigrette*
- Southwest Avocado Chicken Salad
  *without: bacon, cheese, ranch, and dressing/vinaigrette*
- Apple Pecan Chicken Salad
  *without: cheese, cranberries, roasted pecans (if sweetened), and dressing/vinaigrette*
- Chicken Caesar Salad
  *ask for grilled, not crispy chicken*
  *without: crispy chicken, cheese, croutons, and dressing/vinaigrette*

## Sides

- Plain Baked Potato
  *without: cheese, dried cranberries, brown sugar walnuts, bacon, and dressing/vinaigrette*
- Side Caesar Salad
  *without: cheese, croutons, and dressing/vinaigrette*
- Apple Bites

## Breakfast

- Apple Bites

# Whataburger

Drink: Water

<u>Chicken</u>

- Grilled Chicken Sandwich
  *without: white bread (whole wheat/grain or lettuce bun instead), sauce, and cheese*

<u>Burgers</u>

*without cheese, mustard, and white bread (whole wheat/grain or lettuce bun instead)*

- Whataburger
- Double Meat Whataburger

<u>Sides</u>

*instead of dressing, ask for: lemon, pepper, vinegar, guacamole/avocados, and/or fresh salsa*

- Apple Chicken Salad (with Grilled Chicken)
  *without: cheese, cranberries, and dressing/vinaigrette*
- Garden Salad
  *without: cheese, croutons, and dressing/vinaigrette*
- Apple Bites

Remember:

There's no need to eliminate carbs, starve yourself, have a rigorous meal plan, or count calories! You can have the strength, energy, and positivity provided by delicious healthy food and be fit! The latest medical research shows that losing weight is as simple as not eating products with added sugar and refined grain. We also need lots of vegetables.

# Yard House

Drink: Water

## Snacks

- Guacamole
  *without: chips (ask for soft corn tortillas instead) and feta*
- Chilled Edamame
- Street Tacos A La Carte (Baja Fish, Baja Shrimp, Blackened Shrimp, Asada, or Chipotle Chicken)
  *without: flour tortillas (soft corn tortillas instead), cheese, and sauce (salsa is okay)*
- Ahi Sashimi
  *without soy vinaigrette*
- Chicken Lettuce Wraps
  *without sauce*
- Spicy Tuna Roll (if brown rice is available)
  *without: white rice (brown rice instead) and soy sauce*

## Starter Soups & Salads

*instead of dressing, ask for: lemon, pepper, vinegar, guacamole/avocados, and/or fresh salsa*

- Tomato Bisque
  *without: cheese, dried cranberries, and dressing/vinaigrette*
- Traditional Caesar
  *without: Parmesan crisps, croutons, and Caesar dressing*
- Kale Caesar
  *without: raisins, Parmesan crisps, croutons, and Caesar dressing*
- Chopped Salad
  *without: bacon and dressing/vinaigrette*
- Mixed Field Greens
  *without: croutons and dressing/vinaigrette*

# Yard House (2)

Drink: Water or Low-Fat Milk

## Entrée Salads

*instead of dressing, ask for: lemon, pepper, vinegar, guacamole/avocados, and/or fresh salsa*

- Chicken Kale Caesar (Chicken, Shrimp, Skirt Steak, Salmon, or Ahi)
  *without: raisins, Parmesan crisps, croutons, and Caesar dressing*
- Cobb Salad (Chicken, Shrimp, Skirt Steak, or Salmon)
  *without: cheese, bacon, and dressing/vinaigrette*
- Red Quinoa Salad
  *without: cheese and dressing/vinaigrette*

## House Favorites

- Chicken Enchilada Stack
  *without: cheese, sour cream, and rice (more beans without cheese or brown rice instead)*
- Poke Bowl
  *without: crispy rice, crispy wonton, soy vinaigrette, and sriracha aïoli*

## Steaks

- Rib Eye
  *without: butter, mashed potatoes (plain baked potato instead), broccoli (fresh or grilled vegetables without dressing instead), and steak sauce*
- Skirt Steak Arrachera
  *without: butter (on steak and corn) and white rice (brown rice or beans without cheese instead)*
- Rib Eye & Shrimp
  *without: butter, steak sauce, mashed potatoes (plain baked potato instead), and broccoli (fresh or grilled vegetables without dressing instead)*

# Yard House (3)

Drink: Water

<u>Seafood</u>

- Pan Seared Ahi
  *ask for Ahi to be seared with little to no oil*
  *without: sauce and white rice (brown rice or more vegetables instead)*
- Mediterranean Salmon
  *without: tahini and raisins*
- Ginger Crusted Salmon
  *without: butter, peanut vinaigrette, and mashed potatoes (plain baked potato instead)*

<u>Street Tacos</u>

*with soft corn tortillas, not flour tortillas*

- Baja Shrimp or Baja Fish
  *without sriracha aïoli*
- Blackened Shrimp
  *without cumin crema*
- Asada
- Chipotle Chicken
  *without: sauce, cheese, and cumin crema*

<u>Burgers</u>

*without white bread bun (lettuce, whole wheat/grain, or rye bun instead)*

- Beef Burger
  *without: cheese, sauce, aïoli, and fries (vegetables instead)*
- Turkey Burger
  *without: cheese, aïoli, and fries (vegetables instead)*
- Vegan Burger
  *without: onion bun, sauce, and cheese*
- Lamb Burger
  *without: sauce, cheese, caramelized jalapeño shallot relish, and fries (vegetables instead)*

# Yard House (4)

Drink: Water

<u>Sandwiches</u>

*without white bread. ask for lettuce bun, whole wheat/grain bun, or rye bun instead*

- Grilled Chicken & Avocado Sandwich
  *without: cheese, mayo, and fries (vegetables instead)*
- Roasted Turkey Club
  *without: cheese, bacon, mayo, sourdough, and fries (vegetables instead)*
- Seared Ahi Steak Sandwich
  *ask for Ahi to be seared with little to no oil*
  *without: cheese, caramelized onions (grilled onions instead), aïoli, and fries (vegetables instead)*

Remember:
It's common sense that a calorie is not just a calorie. We should be eating lots of good calories and few bad calories! For example, eating 500 calories of vegetables is much healthier than eating 100 calories of a donut.

# Zaxby's

- Drink: Water

<u>Zalads</u>

*instead of dressing, ask for: lemon, pepper, vinegar, guacamole/avocados, and/or fresh salsa*

- The House (Grilled Chicken)
  *without: cheese, fried onions, dressing/vinaigrette, and white bread toast (whole wheat/grain toast instead, if available)*
- The Cobb (Grilled Chicken)
  *without: cheese, bacon, fried onions, dressing/vinaigrette, and white bread toast (whole wheat/grain toast instead, if available)*
- The Caesar
  *without: cheese, bacon, croutons, dressing/vinaigrette, and white bread toast (whole wheat/grain toast instead, if available)*

<u>Sides & Extras</u>

- Basket of Celery
  *without dressing/sauce*
- Side Salad
  *without: cheese, croutons, and dressing/vinaigrette*

> Remember:
> Carry this book with you to help you choose a restaurant, order, and eat out healthily.

# Zoës Kitchen

Drink: Water

## Starters

- Mediterranean Lamb Kafta
  *without: tzatziki and harissa*

## Soups & Salads

*instead of dressing, ask for: lemon, pepper, vinegar, guacamole/avocados, and/or fresh salsa*

- Chicken & Orzo Soup
  *without orzo*
- Mediterranean Lentil Soup
  *without: cheese, croutons, and dressing/vinaigrette*
- Live Med Salad
  *without: Parmesan cheese and dressing/vinaigrette*
- Quinoa Salad
  *without: feta and dressing/vinaigrette*
- Greek Salad
  *without: feta, potato salad, and pita bread*
- Tossed Greek Salad
  *without: pasta salad, caramelized onions (grilled onions instead), feta, dressing/vinaigrette, and pita*

## Sandwiches

- Turkey Stack
  *without: sourdough (7-grain or rye bread instead), feta spread, and rosemary oil*
- Steak Stack
  *without: sourdough (7-grain or rye bread instead), feta spread, and rosemary oil*

# Zoës Kitchen (2)

Drink: Water

<u>Kabobs</u>

- Chicken Kabobs
  *without: feta, oil, and dressing/vinaigrette on salad*
- Steak Kabobs
  *without: Italian salsa verde and feta, oil, and dressing/vinaigrette on salad*
- Salmon Kabobs
  *without: Moroccan harissa and feta, oil, and dressing/vinaigrette on salad*
- Shrimp Kabobs
  *without: tzatziki and feta, oil, and dressing/vinaigrette on salad*

<u>Bowls & Classics</u>

- Cauliflower Rice Bowl
  *without: feta, tzatziki, Israeli skhug, oil, and dressing/vinaigrette*
- Power Grain Bowl
  *without: tzatziki, Moroccan harissa, Mediterranean relish, oil, and dressing/vinaigrette*
- Mediterranean Salad Trio Bowl
  *without: pesto farro (plain farro instead), tzatziki, Italian salsa verde, feta, oil, and dressing/vinaigrette*
- Mediterranean Chicken
  *without: caramelized onions and feta, oil, and dressing/vinaigrette on salad*

# Zoës Kitchen (3)

Drink: Water

## Family Dinners

- Moroccan Chicken Family Dinner
  *without: white rice (cauliflower rice instead), feta, oil, and dressing/vinaigrette on salad*
- Kabob Family Dinner
  *without: sauce, feta, oil, and dressing/vinaigrette on salad*
- Mediterranean Chicken Family Dinner
  *without: caramelized onions (grilled onions instead), feta, oil, and dressing/vinaigrette on salad*

## Sides & Snack Boxes

- Seasonal Fresh Fruit
  *without: feta, tzatziki, Israeli skhug, oil, and dressing/vinaigrette*
- Side Quinoa Salad
  *without: feta and dressing/vinaigrette*
- Roasted Vegetables
  *without: tzatziki, Moroccan harissa, Mediterranean relish, oil, and dressing/vinaigrette*
- Power Grains
  *without: white rice (brown rice instead, if available)*
- Greek Salad
  *without: feta, potato salad, and pita bread*

26109955R00093

Made in the USA
San Bernardino, CA
17 February 2019